# Guide on how to seduce women

*TIPS AND EXAMPLES ON HOW TO GET A GIRLFRIEND, EVEN IF YOU'RE SHY AND AWKWARD.*

*Lilly De*

Copyright © 2021

# 1. INDEX

1. Index .................................................................................................2
2. Child's play... For adults!...................................................................4
   What women can you pick up?.........................................................9
3. What is it that women like in a man?................................................21
   Be relaxed ....................................................................................30
   Knowing how to dress...................................................................32
4. Where to meet women? ....................................................................33
   In the street ..................................................................................33
   On the bus, the subway... .............................................................33
   In a restaurant..............................................................................34
   Supermarket .................................................................................36
   Stores ...........................................................................................36
   Museums ......................................................................................37
   Courses and schools.....................................................................38
   The beach.....................................................................................39
   Parks.............................................................................................39
   Clubs, discos................................................................................39
   Everywhere... ...............................................................................40
5. The first contact................................................................................41
6. What do we say next? .......................................................................51
   The magic of desire ......................................................................52
   Is she the woman in your life? .....................................................53
   It is unique... ................................................................................53
   The art of pleasure........................................................................56
   What to talk about? ......................................................................57

    Being a good listener ..................................................................... 58

    How to conclude? ......................................................................... 60

7.  Advice, thoughts, strategy issues.... ............................................. 62

    Women signals ............................................................................. 63

    You reap what you sow ................................................................. 64

8.  Conclusion ..................................................................................... 66

9.  Bonus: 101 ROMANTIC IDEAS ....................................................... 67

## 2. Child's play... For adults!

Why write a book on this topic? Isn't seduction a natural talent, something you have in your blood, once and for all, or not? That we will never have?

Well, imagine not! Seduction is something that can be learned, like music! Besides, if, as I hope, you apply the few (foolproof) secrets contained in this little book (an indispensable vademecum), you'll soon realize it.

I speak from experience. Because I'm far from a natural charmer. I'm not a millionaire. Far from it. I can't say I'm comfortable. I don't drive a Jaguar or a Ferrari. No, only in a modest Renault. My salary would hardly allow me another car, since I'm just a modest freelance journalist. I write articles for various magazines and newspapers, which I don't always sign. And I supplement my income by translating American works.

So nothing to become famous and attract women, because, as everyone knows, fame is undoubtedly one of the safest aphrodisiacs for women. But I don't have this weapon, since my job, as you may have guessed, is pretty obscure.

I don't even have the body of Robert Redford or Alain Delon. I'm not that good looking. I'm pretty ordinary. There's nothing particularly interesting about me.

Yet I must say that I have had extraordinary success with women. So much so that (and I say this without any pretense) I'm almost spoiled for choice when it comes to deciding who to spend the evening or night with.

I can also say, for those who are interested, that you can meet at least one new woman a day. Does that leave you skeptical? Does it seem unbelievable to you?

I too, just two years ago, would have been skeptical if I had heard such a statement. More importantly, I could never have believed it could be applied to me. To others perhaps, in a time of crisis. But to me, who by the time I was twenty-five had had only two rather brief relationships and who was not sickly shy, but very shy, even if I was able to control it....

No, you shouldn't have dreamed in color.... Women didn't like me for years and probably wouldn't for years to come. Since most of my friends were in relationships, I became increasingly reclusive. I was no longer invited to parties or dinners because I had become the fifth wheel....

Needless to say, I was bored out of my mind and had come to hope for some kind of miracle. For example, that my soulmate would one day come ringing the doorbell of my apartment and throw herself into my arms to make a big declaration of love to me. Of course, this didn't happen, miracles are not common, in Paris anyway.

Yet, in the past two years, much water has passed under the bridge and many women have passed into my arms. How many women does that mean, you might ask? Do you want figures? Well, let's say a good thirty, which probably isn't a lot if you compare me to Casanova, but it's still remarkable when you consider that since the beginning of my love life I had only known two women.

And I would add that among this 30 or so women, some were literally superb, beautiful as actresses or models. There were some less spectacular ones, I agree, but after all, I repeat, my name is not Alain Delon.

How did this happen to me? To what do I owe this metamorphosis, this surprising change in the course of my amorous destiny? I'll tell you right now that I didn't receive an inheritance from an old aunt, that I didn't win the Goncourt and that I didn't hand over my uncertain physiognomy to a plastic surgeon. No, it all happened by accident. Or maybe it was fate. Whatever. Let me tell you the story, which is very simple.

It was two years ago then, and I got a call one Monday morning from a publisher who needed a translator. It was another publisher who, having been satisfied with my services, had passed on my name. I made an appointment with the publisher who was doing the translations. And I went to his office the day after tomorrow. He immediately appeared extremely friendly.

There was something about his personality, a kind of fluidity that was extremely seductive. Moreover, I wasn't the only one who was susceptible to his charm, as all the women who passed by his office during the half hour he gave me seemed to be subdued. The secretary, a beautiful brunette, the production manager, a shapely blonde Swedish type, and one of his co-workers who had to work out some translation details with me, a redhead with blue eyes.

Yet, when I took advantage of the fact that the director was talking to his colleague, examined him more closely, I realized that if I overlooked his charm, his magnetism, if I considered only his features separately, there was nothing exceptional about him.

Even so, he had some rather serious flaws, the most visible of which was undoubtedly his nose, not as spectacular as Cyrano's, but still quite strong. His forehead was rather bald and he was not particularly tall, nor athletic, although he started out very thin. I must say, though, that mysteriously he had an expression of great elegance.

One thing that was remarkable about him, however, was the brightness of his eyes, blue and glowing. And his smile. An extremely captivating smile. A smile that revealed very ordinary and imperfectly regular teeth, but that seemed to say that its owner was genuinely happy to find you standing there in front of him.

What happened was that the editor, who entrusted me that very day with the translation of a great American novel, took a liking to me. I had the opportunity to see him again and have a drink with him.

I found that his charm was a hit everywhere, not only with his co-workers, but with foreign women who could not be seduced by the fact that he was a publishing executive. As we quickly became more familiar, I asked him why he made such an impression on women.

He first let out a loud laugh, then shrugged and said, "It's the easiest thing in the world."

And he emptied his globe of red in one gulp. That didn't tell me much.

Women love to be beaten," he added, after wiping his lips.

- But you need to know how? I said.

I think he read a certain sadness in my eyes, a certain spite. Then he told me a surprising confidence.

- Would you believe me if I told you that just five years ago I couldn't get a girlfriend out of a hundred tries?

The surprise on my face amused him. It was like I was telling him he was bluffing, that he wasn't serious.

- It's the absolute truth," he said.

Trust calls trust, I confessed to him that I was currently in this situation and that I was sorry for it. After all, I wasn't that bad, I was relatively smart, I was well enough to do translations, and without being overly confident, I wasn't cloyingly shy. I could bet a woman without trembling.

- If you can talk to a woman, you can do anything. I didn't get that. Nothing? What did he mean?

- That's the main thing," he explained. It's the foundation.

That night I had a conversation, or rather a lesson in seduction, that would change my life, not just my love life, but my whole life, because the confidence that comes from pleasing women gives a more general confidence, a self-confidence that I personally had never known or even suspected until then.

After promising him that I wouldn't use his techniques to play on his courts, he told me all of his secrets. I was amazed at their simplicity and logic.

This fascinating filmmaker recently died in a car accident. It is for this reason, in his memory, as a posthumous thank you, that I have decided to write down the secrets he confided in me. He did me so much good that I feel it is my duty to do the same, so that as many men as possible (and, likewise, women) can benefit from the advice he gave me. I think if he were still alive, he would be happy with this initiative.... As long as no one comes to play on his fields!

Before I get into the heart of the matter (and I must admit that I feel an impatient flicker in my pen that seems very promising, because in order to illustrate the principles I have learned, I will have to resort to real-life examples whose memory still moves me), before I get into the heart of the matter, then, I must make a small point.

The purpose of this book is not to make you one of those pickup artists who become as alienated and unhappy with their obsession with seduction as those who, on the other hand, fail to please women. I have no objection to the reader using the secrets in this book to own a new woman every day.

But that's not what it's about. What I'm trying to do is help men who, for one reason or another, don't meet women or who have had successive failures with them (as unfortunately happened to me until two years ago), to break the cycle of their loneliness.

I want to promote connection between men and women. Because there's nothing more natural. By the way, remember that making first contact with a woman doesn't necessarily mean sleeping with her that night.

There could be so much more at the end of the line. A wonderful friendship. Mutual tenderness. A contact that could benefit you professionally. A simple exchange of ideas that will allow you to have a pleasant evening and grow socially. And who knows, maybe, eventually, there's even love. True love, the one that most people are looking for.

Unfortunately, all too often in life there are missed opportunities, encounters that never happen, simply because of us. For that woman you met yesterday on the street, that absolutely beautiful woman you shyly followed from afar and didn't dare approach despite perhaps a subtle smile of encouragement, who knows, maybe she was the woman of your life, with whom you could have had a great love story. Maybe she was a woman you would have a wonderful relationship with. And you might never see her again.

It is infinitely better to feel remorse for being rejected than to feel regret for not trying. At least in the first case, you'll have a clear conscience. And maybe even a bargain of the heart....

Yet, nothing is easier than seducing a woman, or flirting as we say today. When you know how to do it. And that's what I intend to show you.

You too will soon say, as I did, that this is a child's game, for adults. If someone as fundamentally ordinary as me has managed to make many achievements in the time it takes to say that, there is absolutely no reason why you can't do the same.

## WHAT WOMEN CAN YOU PICK UP?

This is a fundamental question that I hasten to answer. Simple. All women. No matter their age or status. Rich or poor. Famous or completely unknown. Teachers, nurses, salesclerks, typists. Single, divorced, etc. I'm not just saying this to encourage you. It's the absolute truth.

I have to tell you something: times have changed a lot in the last twenty years. Not so long ago, it was rare for a woman to make love before getting married. Those that did, did so very discreetly and did not make a show of it.

They didn't and risked getting a bad reputation.... Now most women start having sex at a very young age and don't bother to marry their lover.

Many women are freedom-loving and don't want to make a real commitment, preferring to invest most of their energy in pursuing a career. Most modern women are financially independent, which makes them free in many ways, including physically.

And then, the arrival of the contraceptive pill has greatly reduced if not completely eliminated the fear of unwanted pregnancy. In many ways, then, women are now more free. And more available. And, just like men, they seek love every day.

In this regard, I would like to mention the movie novel that was based on this wonderful film by the late François Truffaut: The Man Who Loved Women. Also, if there was a movie I could recommend to put you in the right frame of mind to show you that it is easy to pick up women and that a very ordinary looking man can make almost daily conquests, I would point you to this movie without hesitation.

If you haven't had a chance to see it, it is, as the title suggests, the story of one man, Bertrand Morane, an engineer by profession and a bachelor by trade, whose only passion in life is women. Women. All women.

The imagination and ingenuity with which he achieves his goals is admirable. And the results are also admirable, despite some inevitable failures. One day, he decides to write down his memories of love, to make a ro- man of sorts. At some point, he wonders, fascinated by the tide of women who, in the spring, pour into the streets of Montpellier, where he is.

There are thousands of them, every day, walking the streets.... But who are all these women? Where are they going? To what appointment? If their hearts are free, then their bodies are up for grabs, and it seems to me that I have no right to let the opportunity pass.

I'll tell you the truth: they want the same thing I want, they want love. Everyone wants love. All kinds of love. Physical love and sentimental love, or even just the selfless tenderness of someone who has chosen someone else for life and is no longer looking at anyone. I'm not there, I'm looking at everyone.

However, even though most women think about love on a daily basis and enjoy being tested, they may not admit it. They may be cold and reluctant at first. Most live in fear of being seen as easy. They don't hate it when men take a little trouble before giving them their last favors. But there's one important thing you should remember that will remove all your hesitations and fears: not only are all women willing to be beaten, they love it.

In fact, the best evidence of this is that the opposite worries and depresses them. Women are always happy to say at the end of the day that they were approached by a stranger who charmed them or that a man invited them for a drink or offered them a ride.

They may not openly admit that they were 'hit on,' as the term is overused and abhorrent to some women. They will say that they met someone by chance, that a man offered to carry their shopping bag, that he helped them park their car. All perfectly innocent things on the surface. It's just a matter of nomenclature. But in most cases, of course, the man who offered to carry a heavy bag for the woman was simply hitting on her. Very politely, very civilly, but he was hitting on her just the same.

In fact, sometimes it's surprising how easy it is to seduce a woman. Even a woman who not only doesn't look free, but actually isn't. Let me share a little anecdote with you. Since this is a true story (and in this case of the author of these pages), you'll understand that the names I'll mention are fictitious. I don't care about my own reputation, but there are those of others....

For six months, after completing the translation of the American novel entrusted to me by the man to whom I owe the secrets I am sharing with you, I worked at the publishing house, doing various editorial jobs. I was given a small office that suited me perfectly. The door opened onto one of the busiest hallways of the publishing house, so I could see all the women who worked there. And there were a lot of them. And pretty cute, too.

One day, one of them, whom I had noticed, was appointed as the new secretary in the department where I worked. She wasn't Catherine Deneuve, but she was pretty. Above all, she was very sexy.

She was a rather skinny brunette with a waspish waist and fiery eyes. She also had an outrageous way of smoking a cigarette. It was breathtaking. If it weren't between us, between men, I wouldn't tell you the way she walked. Always wearing stilettos (probably to make herself taller), she had a way of swaying her hips that literally infuriated other women, but delighted men.... Men rarely escape certain effects, even if they are ostentatiously inflated.

Long story short, let's say a friend of mine came to the publishing house one day and hit me. We've known each other for 20 years and he's been hitting me for 20 years. When we were younger, it was over cigarettes or other trinkets. Now it's for more serious reasons. But, because he is a childhood friend, I don't refuse him anything. When he came to my office he was very excited and immediately explained why. When he arrived he had followed a woman who was wiggling in an extraordinary way. This woman, as you may have guessed, was none other than the new secretary whom for convenience I will call Ginette. She had obviously preceded him into the office.

This childhood friend, whose name was Jean, was going through a rather dark period, emotionally. He was separating from his wife and for a few weeks, having not yet found a new apartment, he had been accepting the hospitality of friends when he wasn't sleeping in a hotel. He immediately asked me to tell him who this hot secretary was. A new one, I explained. Is there something going on between you?

No," I replied and was about to add, "Not yet. But he wouldn't let me finish.

- So you definitely need to introduce me to her.

Friends first, right? That's what I thought, anyway. On my way out of the office, I was going to introduce him to Ginette, but she was on her way out too, so they crossed paths and saw each other for a split second. A split second, I say. You'll soon understand the consequences.

Disappointed, my friend Jean, who by the way is not too ugly, and proudly sports a Gallic mustache of which he is very proud (and rightly so, because it has earned him a lot of success with women, and we'll come back to that in another chapter), my friend Jean, begged me to arrange something, to arrange a meeting between Ginette and him. What wouldn't we do for our friends?

The next day, I was playing matchmaker with the hottest girl in the department. I had a few regrets. Shouldn't I think about myself, be a little more selfish? I promise. I only have one word... However, chatting with Ginette the next morning during a coffee break, I told her that my friend had been very impressed with her and hadn't stopped talking about her since he'd seen her the day before.

- He would love to meet you," I said. She looked confused by what I had just said. I must say I was improvising all sorts of details, coming up with compliments that my friend had never suggested. Too bad, I felt I could have seduced this girl if I had been quicker.

- All she has to do is call me," Ginette replied bluntly. I was stunned. She had agreed to a date with a man she didn't know, hadn't even spoken to, and had only caught a glimpse of.

I also wondered if she would recognize him for sure. My surprise is magnified tenfold when I learn a little later that although she is not officially married, she has been living with a man for two years. A modern woman, no doubt. If I tell you about this adventure in detail, even though it's not mine, it's to show you how much today's women love to be courted, how available they are, and how much they love adventure, probably as much as you do.

When I tell my friend Jean the good news, he rejoices and asks me for a new favor. Would it be too much to ask me to give him my apartment for the night? Why? He doesn't want Ginette to know he's married and getting a divorce. Going to the hotel would immediately alarm her. Since it's a good cause, I can't refuse.

The next day he calls Ginette at the office and makes an appointment with her. They are going to have dinner together, at a nice little restaurant. Just before he picks her up from the office, he comes over to my place to get the keys and asks me a little anxiously how far she can go the first night. Since I barely know her, I don't dare advise him one way or the other, I just say, "You'll see how things go.

For my part, I contact a friend who kindly gives me hospitality for the night. The next day, my boyfriend tells me everything, overjoyed. She herself took the initiative. At one point, in the restaurant, she told him candidly:

- Can I ask you something? - Yes, you can.

- Kiss me...

Needless to say, the night was over. Their romance didn't last. Ginette soon found out. In a very simple way. When she handed me my paycheck one Thursday, she noticed that my address was the same as Jean's. They had a violent argument, followed by a few words of protest. They had a violent argument, followed by a final breakup, but that didn't upset my boyfriend, because he had decided to go back to his wife.

Some time passed. Every time I saw Ginette again - and I saw her several times a day - I thought it was a shame I had been so hesitant. I decided to take a chance. I invited her to dinner. She accepted. Throughout the evening I was nothing but friendly, especially since she mentioned her partner two or three times, which didn't fail to cool me down. But as I walked her to her car, at the last moment, in greeting her, I ventured to kiss her and soon parted my lips. To my surprise, she didn't push me away. Not immediately. In fact, after a fairly long kiss, she pulled up and said, angrily:

- I knew it. You men are all the same, you only have one idea in mind.

I stammered out an explanation, accompanied by compliments, which you should never fail to do.

- Well, I... I'm sorry... I didn't mean to, but you're so beautiful, so sensual... I couldn't help it... I couldn't help it...

I immediately saw her anger fall away. Like she was spellbound. In short, I told her that she had put me off, that I was not responsible for my actions. I anticipate here to tell you that this usually has a devastating effect on women. They hate cold seducers who never get excited. I would even say, and this is what my personal experience has shown me, that the surest way to disturb a woman is to be disturbed yourself.

If you are not sincerely disturbed (which is ideal, since emotion gives us eloquence, if not verbally, then in another, more mysterious, invisible way, to which I will return later), if you are not truly disturbed, then pretend to be. However, in the case that occupied me that evening, these fine words were not enough to temper Ginette's anger for long. She soon returned to the charge, her beautiful eyes flashing with vengeance.

Jean told you how I kissed and you wanted to compare.... Who do you think I am? You think I'm going to sleep with the whole gang?

He wasn't wrong. Jean had described to me in such detail the wild nights he had spent in Ginette's arms that naturally I was envious. It only confirmed what I already thought of her, that she was an extremely sensual woman. But of course I had to deny everything. I didn't laugh about it too much. But Ginette gave me a cold shower when she said:

- I want you to know one thing. I will never go back to your apartment. And I will never sleep with you.

I didn't protest. I didn't even tease her. I simply shrugged my shoulders and acted like a gentleman. This is a strategy you should use on almost every occasion, though.

Let me make a brief aside here that fits well with my anecdote. You're in a bar and you're hitting on a woman. She rejects you. You don't need to start insulting her. You don't need to tell her that she's nothing but a good-for-nothing. A constipated woman. A frigid woman. A lesbian. It won't do you any good. Even if she does.

You don't know anything about this woman. She may have very good reasons for rejecting you. She may have just broken up with her boyfriend and is not in the mood for jokes. She may have just lost her mother to horrible cancer. This is no laughing matter.

Maybe she's simply waiting for someone. Another night you might see her again. Maybe in a better mood. Since you've already approached her, the second meeting will be easier. Besides, even if she's not really interested, it might be the second time with a girl who will succumb to your charms.

With Ginette, I told myself my chances were nil. I was being a little cheeky. It was normal, after all, that she would not throw herself into my arms after being seduced by my best friend and discovering a deception in which I was an accomplice anyway. The next morning, when I saw her again, I simply told her, very amicably:

- Despite what happened yesterday, it would be nice if we went out for a drink one night as friends.

- Maybe so.

- I'll leave you my phone number, just in case.

A week later, to my surprise, she used that number one night. To go for a drink. It was a nice night. Ginette drank a lot. But she wasn't particularly friendly. I was in a quandary. I was madly in love with her, found her infinitely desirable. That evening she wore a blouse with the top buttons undone. This allowed her beautiful breasts to be seen.

Was she doing it on purpose? If she just wants to be friends, why did she dress so provocatively? Maybe she's just teasing. She wants to show me off. When it came time to walk her to her car, like the first night, my dilemma reached a sort of climax.

I wanted her badly, but at the same time I was afraid of another rejection. Fortunately, I didn't have to decide my dilemma. When I came to place a purely friendly kiss on Ginette's lips, this time she opened her mouth and literally threw herself into my arms. It was a long, passionate kiss.

- Let's smoke a cigarette in the car," he suggested, no doubt afraid of making a spectacle of himself to casual passersby, despite the relatively late hour.

Of course, I didn't object. In the car, it was an even more passionate kiss. I allowed myself to be more daring. But the comfort of my Renault being somewhat limited in this respect, we went to my apartment where the night seemed very short. In the morning, Ginette asked me with admirable candor, a girlish air that delighted me:

- What must you think of me?

That you are the most passionate woman I have ever met. But what do you think of me?

I guess I'm an easy man," I replied before letting her gamble, having guessed what she probably expected me to say.

Joker... she said amused.

It was more or less a joke. Because I believe that today the expression easy woman has no meaning anymore and should make people smile as much as the expression easy man. Both men and women feel the same pleasure in each other's arms. And isn't it often the woman who insidiously sets a trap for the man? The man who believes that the woman has fallen into his trap is often mistaken.

Women are more adept at this kind of story than we usually think. In this case, wasn't it Ginette who led me on, so to speak? Of course it was me who gave her my phone number. She also knew I was interested in her, my failed attempt to seduce her being proof of that. But she was still the one who had called me. More importantly, she was the one who started the ball rolling. As I left my apartment that morning, Ginette said, in a tone that was half serious, half mean:

- I swore to myself that I would never set foot in this place again.

- These are the circumstances of life," I said in a tone devoid of mockery.

But the first thought that came to my mind was the old maxim, "Never say, fountain, I will not drink of your water..."

To close this story, I eventually had a relationship with Ginette that lasted a few months and ended when she left her job to go work in Lyon, where she had decided to follow her partner. She had never taken me seriously. Our separation was as amicable as possible.

The reason I have told this anecdote is that, in addition to the pleasure I derive from its evocation, I consider it highly instructive.

illustrates a principle. Most women seek adventure. Even those who are seemingly unattainable. It also shows that you shouldn't take a woman's rejection completely seriously, no matter how emphatic.

A "no", even a very convinced one, can quickly turn into an exhilarating "yes". Female desire is something infinitely capricious. In both directions. Nothing can set it off. Nothing can make it die. Why did Ginette change her mind about me? Do you know what I think? Since you can't answer me, of course, I'll do it for you. Maybe Ginette never really changed her mind about me. Maybe she always liked me. She didn't want to be seen as an easy woman, especially after what happened to her with my boyfriend Jean. She was playing a game.

This story also demonstrates another principle that I will return to later. It's about insistence, perseverance, and especially its counterbalance. We will see later that sometimes it is very effective to be persistent.

But sometimes you have to make a strategic retreat, taking one step back so you can take two steps forward. This can have a tremendous effect. The woman was flattered by your first assault. But she refused to give in to your advances. This is very good. You're not sorry. You are cool, relaxed, etc. You let her know that it's not the end of the world, that it won't kill you, that you'll still find her likable. This is what happens very often, I have experienced it myself on many occasions. The woman has been flattered by your courtship. Now you do nothing. You are in a frenzy. She often starts to wonder.

Your friendly neutrality annoys her. Maybe he really doesn't like me, she thinks. Why did he stop so soon? This may seem absolutely contradictory, since he just told you he'd rather you stop trying. But here's the thing.

Desire is probably the most contradictory thing in the world. Often the woman will try to grab you, not to let go. She will want to take you back. Let her. She is likely to be much more skilled than you and will quickly achieve her goals, which by an incredible coincidence are also yours. We'll talk about this later.

Remember this. When you want to flirt, don't exclude any woman outright. You won't seduce all of them, because the attraction has to be mutual. But you'd be foolish not to try your luck. Even women who seem to be emotionally happy and who, by definition, should be hard conquests, are susceptible to seduction. Think of Madame Bovary, too. How many women are like her, even today. The streets are full of Emma Bovarys. It's up to you to play the right card.

There is one more thing you should consider that most men never think about, precisely because they are men. Not only do women love to be tried, but many of them have told me that they wish men would try them more. Not only is it in a woman's nature to please, with all her clothes and tricks geared towards that end, but from their upbringing they are generally condemned to not being able to make the first move and waiting for the man to do it. They also fall in love at first sight, on the street, in a bar, on the bus, etc., and their greatest desire, when they see a man they like, is for him to hit on them.

On that note, I'd like to mention again the film novel The Man Who Loved Women, which I highly recommend you read. It can only enlighten you about the amorous mores of our century and about women. This is Geneviève speaking, the one who will edit the novel of Bertrand, the hero. They have recently become lovers and are chatting in bed:

- 'But still,' says Geneviève, 'there is one thing I disagree with, and that is when you write (I don't remember exactly) 'Women think about love in a more general way than men. ' I assure you that we too have our curiosities, our sudden desires. Now I can tell you that the first time I felt like you was in the Paris office when you were talking to the layout artist. I remember very well: it was very hot and at one point you took off your sweater and had a cigarette in your mouth. You were so absorbed in the conversation that you did everything mechanically. So you took off your sweater like that, pulling the collar, without even taking the cigarette out of your mouth! Well, suddenly, because of that, I felt like making love to you!"

The reason I allowed myself such a long quote is because it contains valuable lessons. The sympathetic editor confirms that women can have the same lives as men. He also gives further proof of the capriciousness of desire, which can arise at the slightest pretext. It also gives us information about one of the most important aspects of seducing women, which we will talk about right away. She did not tell Bertrand Morane that he seduced her because he had a muscular torso, an Apollo-like profile, or because he was tall. Moreover, the hero of the film, played by Charles Denner, has none of these attributes. Geneviève tells him that she wanted to make love to him because of his intensity, because he was so absorbed that he didn't think about taking out his cigarette when he took off his sweater. This is a very important indication.

# 3. WHAT IS IT THAT WOMEN LIKE IN A MAN?

This is what I was getting at, as you may have already guessed. Many men are afraid to approach women because they don't think they are good looking enough. This is very sad. Because fortunately for us men, women are much less superficial. Men are generally very attracted to physical appearance, facial beauty, breasts, legs. A survey was conducted in the United States of 3,000 women. The question these women were asked was, "What is it about a man that attracts you in the first place?

Surprisingly, the majority responded with personality.

The second most important aspect is the eyes and figure.

Then, even more surprising (but not so much if you admit that women have the same sexual mindset as men), buttocks.

The vast majority don't even mention the fact that the man must be seven feet tall, have big blue eyes, be a consummate athlete and drive a Jaguar, and of course constantly travel the world as CEO of a multinational corporation. This, you'll agree, is an undeniable advantage.

Men should stop having complexes and fearing the trade of women, because, for example, they have

their noses a little too long, or turned upwards, because they don't think they're tall enough, their skin isn't perfect, or they're obsessed with starting to go bald.

What women like in a man is his entire personality, the way he moves, the way he talks, that indefinable thing called charm. It is generally believed that charm is something natural that you are born with, in greater or lesser doses. It is true that some people are born with extraordinary natural charm.

There are famous examples, the most illustrious of which is probably Rudolph Valentino. One must keep in mind, however, that the appeal of some movie stars is partly manufactured, if not fabricated, and that women often succumb to it from afar, and in advance, without ever having met their idol.

However, one thing is certain, contrary to what is generally believed, charm can be acquired, thanks to special and secret techniques that I will indicate to you in the following chapters. These techniques, if you at least practice them seriously for half an hour a day, will give us a special grace, a kind of eerie magnetic aura that acts not only on women but also on men.

These techniques were passed on to me by my editor friend who had practiced them and changed his life through them. The confidence, the trust, the presence to others and in the moment, the strength of concentration they give us can transform your life. But let's not get ahead of ourselves, I'll come back to this topic later.

The personality, the overall image that a man projects is therefore far more decisive than plastic beauty in pleasing women. I will borrow an amusing anecdote from film history to illustrate my point. In his early days, long before he became famous, Jean-Louis Trintignant was asked by Brigitte Bardot to play a young leading role opposite her.

The first reaction of the blonde starlet, who had already begun to torment the minds of men, was categorical. There was no way she was going to act next to this good-for-nothing actor, whom she thought was horrible, and in any case absolutely unworthy of playing the young leading man, especially next to her. The director, however, held firm and imposed Trintignant. Brigitte Bardot was annoyed and had to take her side. But a surprising metamorphosis took place. After two weeks, Bardot was madly in love with Trintignant and they had a passionate affair.

What had happened to bring about such a change? I can see nothing but the effect of charm. It should be noted that Jean-Louis Trintignant subsequently won the hearts of thousands of French women who found him extremely charming. Of course, this is where the phenomenon of fame comes into play. Fame, power and wealth are powerful aphrodisiacs for women.

Fortunately, they are not necessary for their conquest. I am living proof of that. I have none of these attributes. Yet, in the past two years, as I've told you, I haven't counted my successes with women. There are several men in my situation. And soon, no doubt, you will join our ranks. It's up to you.

Anecdotes like the one I just told about Jean-Louis Trintignant and Brigitte Bardot are common in film history. Jean-Paul Belmondo was in the same situation as Trintignant when he started out in film. When he started, no one would have thought that one day he would be able to play the roles of a young leading man.

Many also tried to discourage him from pursuing a career in film. He was small, rather puny at the time, and was even considered ugly. Yet within a few years he would become a true sex symbol. Women may never find him handsome, but they think he has a face, as they say. Belmondo is the eternal optimist, the fighter.

And he's also a smile. And of course he's a great speaker. He always has the right word, the right answer. He seems to be saying, let those who love me follow me. His formula has worked. He had beautiful companions like Raquel Welch. For a skinny guy who was considered too ugly to be in movies, he didn't do too badly.

Other examples? There are many. Did you know, for example, that Woody Allen is considered one of the most important "sex symbols" in the United States? He even surpasses actors like Robert Redford in the love ratings of American women. Yet, if anyone has an unattractive physique, it's him. In terms of classic beauty, with his sad little eyes that aren't graced by his heavy glasses, his already noticeably receding forehead, and his skinny body, he's way behind Jean-Louis Trintignant and Jean- Paul Belmondo. Both have at least a sporty appearance and a certain vitality. Woody Allen looks like a neurasthenic and admits to being depressed most of the time, consoling himself with the fact that this is when he is funniest and finds his best banter.

But imagine the possibilities it leaves you with. If Woody Allen has managed, probably despite himself, to become a sex symbol, if thousands of probably very beautiful and sexy women dream of having him in their bed, then anyone can successfully flirt. Sure, you could say he's famous, a millionaire and a director, which gets him many young starlets hoping for roles in his films. And some, myself included, consider him a genius. His humor is irresistible on screen and no doubt with women.

Humor is one of the surest resources for seducing women. 'If you can make a woman laugh,' said Stendhal, 'she is already half in your bed. "But it's far from beautiful. He's barely drinkable. And he has become a sex symbol.

Today's beauty standards have changed drastically. In the case of classical beauty, perfect regularity of features is no longer an absolute criterion. I borrow many examples from cinema because the Seventh Art really conveys, and sometimes even models, the values of society. Since the New Wave of the 1960s, we have seen the appearance of faces that are basically quite ordinary, everyday heroes, who nevertheless managed to seduce millions of viewers. On the male side, I mentioned Trintignant and Belmondo, Woody Allen. There are many others. In the United States, for example, Dustin Hoffman. Al Pacino. On the female side: Annie Girardot, Jeanne Moreau, Isabelle Hupert, Fanny Ardant, Liza Minelli, Barbara Streisand. The list could go on and on. These faces are not only quite ordinary, but they often come with notable flaws that sometimes only add to their charm.

Speaking of flaws, there's a famous one you all know. Cleopatra's nose. If it had been different, Pasquale said, the course of the world would have been changed. But even if it had been more perfect, Cleopatra's life probably wouldn't have changed. Contrary to popular belief, Cleopatra was not a woman of great beauty. Her appearance itself was not remarkable, or at least not impressive, and no doubt many of her contemporaries were prettier than she was. But historians report that Cleopatra possessed qualities that transcended physical beauty. The touch of her presence, if you lived with her, was absolutely irresistible. Her attraction to people, the charm of her conversation, the sound of her voice, and the way she moved were fascinating.

How often do you hear someone, man or woman, say, "He (or she) isn't particularly nice but he (or she) has something." You can get that "something." In fact, you already have it, all of you. It's inside you, more or less deeply buried. Like a hidden power that hasn't manifested. It's up to you to explode it and use it. We'll see later how.

So what matters, much more than plastic beauty, is the total impression, what you give off, which depends on true beauty, inner beauty. You are probably not satisfied with your physical appearance. Don't worry. Most people are unfortunately like you. No reason. You are unique. You can express your beauty, which may be different from the comparisons society has instilled in you, but is no less real.

Also, classic beauty is not necessarily an advantage in itself. Did you know that many women are wary? They may admire a handsome man, but they are often intimidated by too-perfect beauty. They shy away from it. They often associate it with inevitable frivolity and prefer not to get involved with a man who will betray them at the first opportunity. Think about this. It's an advantage. This principle has a corollary, in a way. Many men believe that very beautiful women are unattainable, especially if they themselves are not so beautiful. Well, you'd be surprised how much of a handicap beauty can be for women. Let me give you a case study. A personal experience.

About a year ago, I took a German class for a while. For a long time I dreamed of reading some of the great Germanic philosophers in the original. Incidentally, taking courses in anything is great for dating. I must admit that this thought was not totally unrelated to my decision to take these courses. You have to combine business with pleasure, right?

The first evening I noticed a woman of extraordinary beauty. Long black hair, brown eyes also almost black, a narrow nose, very fine and magnificent teeth, real pearls. Finally, words seemed insufficient.

What confirmed for me the idea that it was extremely beautiful, and will convince you of what I'm saying, is that I wasn't the only one in the room.

I was the only one admiring her. In fact, it didn't take me long to realize that all the men in the class had noticed her and couldn't take their eyes off her. I didn't laugh the first night. I was too impressed. I froze. None of the other male students hit on her. In fact, I noticed that none of the men dared to talk to her, much less sit next to her.

In fact, this woman was always alone. Completely alone. As if no one saw her, even though people kept looking at her. Yet there was nothing haughty or cold about this woman. She seemed very simple, friendly. She often even smiled slightly, almost invitingly, in response to the stares of her admirers.

Remembering the principles my late friend had explained to me, especially the one that by definition all women are accessible, even the most beautiful ones, I decided to try my luck. I had worked out my plan the week before. I sat next to her and left the class fifteen minutes before the end. Ostentatiously. So that she would notice my departure. Now I had an excuse ready. You can use this trick if you have a good idea to sign up for an evening class to meet new people.

Upon entering the classroom, I approached this sublime woman and, explaining that I had to leave the previous class before it ended, asked her if the teacher had said anything important and if she could pass me her notes.

She greeted me with a wide smile, almost as if I were Prince Charming to her, or even a lifeline. Soon I would understand why. She invited me to sit down and handed me her notes with true, unconfessed pleasure. I was in a state of extraordinary excitement. I was even more excited when, after class, she asked me if I wanted to have coffee at her house.

I was almost stuttering. I thought I was dreaming. I knew since

I had just met this beautiful woman for two hours and she invited me to her home for coffee. I accepted with enthusiasm. It went beyond my expectations. Within an hour of arriving at her home, I was in her arms and it wasn't to copy German notes. Then we were completely in each other's arms. After our embrace, I couldn't help but ask her, so amazed was I at my good fortune:

- Why me?

She seemed surprised by my question. She probably hadn't noticed how ordinary I was, how much more beautiful she was than me. I was so surprised that I forgot that even beautiful women don't necessarily look for beauty in men. What this divinely beautiful woman revealed to me stunned me. She told me that I was the first man who had dared to talk to her for a year. I didn't understand.

- I'm not successful with men," she says sadly.

- Yet you are the most beautiful woman I have ever met.

- He asked me with a skepticism that was hardly false modesty, I soon realized.

As surprising as it may seem, this woman wasn't lying. Despite her stunning beauty, she was not a hit with men. Besides, I was a fool, wasn't that what had happened in German class? No doubt all men admired her, loved her from afar, but no one came close to her. Strictly speaking, she was not successful with men. She told me that she had been separated for a year, that her husband had left her for a very ordinary woman whose picture she showed me. She showed me a picture of her, it was actually a friend of hers. She was really ordinary, I could tell. She had something else. No doubt about it. At least in her husband's eyes.

I also had the opportunity at the same time to see her husband. I got another surprise, almost a shock. Her husband was a small, chubby man, almost completely bald. And he had managed to marry a goddess, whom by the way he had left. I hid my surprise, the reasons for which would no doubt have displeased my exquisite mistress. All the same! There was something incredible about it.

And yet, no! It is an unfounded misconception that very beautiful women seek out very handsome men. In fact, they often prefer to have their beauty highlighted by a more ordinary, less conspicuous partner. They are often looking for a minion. It's a role that suits me perfectly.... And probably for you, too. But when you ignore these things, what "beautiful" opportunities you're missing, if I may say so.

I wasn't at the end of my surprises. Suzanne (since that was her name) soon told me that she didn't think she was beautiful, or at least not really beautiful. The only evidence of this was that she wasn't very successful with men. What a strange situation! I couldn't believe my ears. When I started telling her again that she was stunningly beautiful (which I thought very sincerely), she smiled with wonder. She admitted that I was the first man to pay her such a compliment. Yet her beauty was comparable, though different, to Catherine Deneuve's. If that gives you any idea.

My relationship with this woman was unfortunately brief. Her husband returned to her a month after our first night. Her marriage had lasted five years and she was still attached to him. So she decided to move back in together.

This little story is instructive in many ways. The first lesson you should learn from this, in my opinion, is this: Never hesitate to meet a woman simply because she is a woman.

Because she is very beautiful. I would even go so far as to say that, in a way, it's easier to please very beautiful women. You'll say that I'm exaggerating, that I'm exaggerating a bit. But wait. I say this because very beautiful women can inspire you more. If you like them more, you will be more enthusiastic about them, your courtship will be more sincere, your desire will be stronger. And desire is contagious and often irresistible.

You need to keep this other point in mind. Many very beautiful women do not think that they are sincerely beautiful. They are often extremely critical of themselves. They find small flaws in themselves, which they exaggerate. They worry about their own beauty. So they constantly need to be reassured, to be told that they are beautiful, to be reminded of it. That's why you're there. In the future, you should never be afraid to approach a woman you think is too beautiful. Remember that fortune favors the bold.

Speaking of your appearance, there's another point to remember. Like beautiful women, you are generally much harder on yourself than others are. We are often fixated on a particular flaw, while people, when they meet us, only see the whole, are influenced by the overall impression. They see a person. To convince yourself of this, you only have to think about the way you yourself perceive other men or women. You will realize that you usually look at the whole picture, the impression of the whole personality. So why should people behave differently with you?

Although appearance is in some ways secondary, that doesn't mean you should neglect it. There are aspects of your appearance that you have some control over. The American Public Survey of Women's Preferences revealed that most women like a thin man.

This is not surprising. You also have a preference for the thin woman, at least in general. To be thin is to be young. It is a form of elegance that is accessible to almost everyone. In any case, a thin man always looks more elegant to women. If you have a few extra pounds, try to be a little more moderate at the table and exercise more. This will improve your overall appearance. You'll have more energy. More energy. You'll be more positive. Your complexion will go from dull to rosy.

Your eyes will be more radiant. You will feel fresh and happy. Being fit means being stylish. People always admire someone who is in good shape. Exercise is accessible to everyone. Don't be afraid to do it. And sports usually offer excellent opportunities to meet people of the opposite sex.

One last word on food. Remember that Westerners generally eat too much. Twice as much as we should. And unfortunately, we're digging our own graves with our teeth. So reduce the amount you eat. Not only will you be slimmer, which will definitely make you more popular with women, but it will give you a whole new physical impression. Especially if you reduce meat. Choose fish over meat, white meat over red meat, and limit yourself to three or four meat meals a week. Never eat two meat meals a day. You can find your protein in many other foods. A weekly fast, or a juice-only day, also has an excellent effect on the body, both physically and nervously.

Your first charm lesson is this: eat frugally. Your complexion will lighten, you'll feel a new energy flow through your body, your eyes will become brighter, your thinking more vivid. Try it. After only a week you will feel a transformation.

Of course, always keep in mind that your diet should remain balanced, even if it is lighter. Remember that we are what we eat. Eat light, you'll feel light, you'll feel a new good mood come over you, all the time, and your fascination with your surroundings will be increased.

## BE RELAXED

We live in a world of extreme stress and tension. People are in a hurry and nervous. You can gain a lot by practicing relaxation. Take a yoga class or an autogenic training class. Go to www.auto-hypnose.com. Or pick up one of the many books in bookstores. Remember the rare occasions when you met a truly relaxed person. In our fast-paced century, this is something of a balm. A relaxed person always makes a good impression. Their calmness makes you feel confident. You're more sensitive to their arguments, you're more easily convinced. Calmness is in itself a charm and seduces more than you think.

You might argue that your main problem with women is really nervousness or shyness. Well, this can be corrected. Practice relaxation every day, complete relaxation. You'll be surprised how quickly the results will come. By the way, a little tip. If in a particular situation you feel very nervous, try to take ten deep and prolonged breaths. You'll be surprised at the results. Just ten deep breaths. Twenty, if you have the time. This is unheard of.

Swimming is a great way to relax and is a perfect complement to yogic relaxation. Whenever you get a chance, jump into a pool and take a few laps. The massaging and invigorating effect of the water is amazing. It is a complete exercise that has the advantage of not straining any muscle or joint, as unfortunately happens with other sports. Swimming also has an incredible psychological effect. Calming. Don't forget that the first environment you evolved in was aquatic. The womb. Swimming, in a way, brings you back to that ideal environment. Many great men have taken up or are taking up swimming. President Kennedy swam regularly. Napoleon found relaxation in his bathtub.

Of course, a certain nervousness can be attractive to women. Famous fools have seduced many hearts. Just think of Woody Allen, whom we mentioned earlier. But in general, a relaxed person is more attractive and, above all, is more likely to be noticed and appreciated, if only by contrast with those around him.

## KNOWING HOW TO DRESS

It's a detail that men don't think about often enough, but one that women give great importance to, actually much greater than we think. Have you ever fallen in love (that's probably a strong word) or rather been attracted or seduced by a simple detail in a woman's clothing? For example, very elegant pumps? Or well-fitting pants? A simple pair of jeans? Or simply a headband that beautifully encircles a poetic brow? Without a doubt. There is a fetishist in every man who sleeps more or less.

Well, the same goes for women. They typically spend three times as much time as men getting dressed. Think about this. And don't hesitate to pay a little more attention to how you dress. Dress sexy. Do not be afraid to wear flashy colors, extravagant clothes, respecting your personality, of course.

You'll be noticed. You'll be more attractive. Maybe the new boots you buy will win you many conquests. Or maybe it will be a very sporty shirt in bright colors. Don't be afraid to be daring. It pays well.

Women hate men who dress in a boring and overly conventional way. Don't forget that the dress is somehow a reflection of your personality. If you forget this, women don't. In conclusion, remember that flirting is selling something, a product that happens to be you.

Packaging isn't everything, but it is important. Make it attractive. Put all the possibilities on your side. If the product behind the packaging is good, all the better.

# 4. Where to meet women?

Just as all women can in principle be tried, all places are good for making contact. There are therefore countless places to go. Once you've tried it, you'll be amazed at how easy it is to succeed wherever you go.

## In the street

I'm going to start with the street, because that's usually the first place you go when you leave your home or office. Some people will argue that this is not done.... They're wrong. It wasn't done fifty years ago.

Today, it is not only done, but it is very effective. In addition, it has an adventurous and romantic side that women really like. If you see a woman you like on the sidewalk, don't hesitate to approach her. We'll see in the next chapter what you can say to her. If you see her and you like her, smile at her. If she responds, don't hesitate to approach her. If you don't have the courage to approach her on the street, follow her.

Perhaps she will walk into a restaurant or store where it will be easier for you to approach her. I must confess that I have personally made several conquests on the street. Women like the boldness it takes for a man to approach her that way. They often reward you for it.

## On the bus, the subway...

Public transportation is also an excellent place to be. If you see an empty seat next to a beautiful woman, do not hesitate to sit down. After all, you are in a public place. Start a conversation. Ask her where to get off to go to a particular place. If you are waiting for the bus or subway, in the same queue, do not hesitate to break the ice.

Check your watch as if you are in a hurry or late. Ask the woman if she thinks the bus or subway will take a long time to arrive. Use this opportunity to compliment her. Tell her that waiting with her is less boring, that you are lucky to find someone as charming as she is. Ask her for information.

## IN A RESTAURANT

Restaurants are also great places to meet. Especially at lunchtime. You may have already noticed that many women eat lunch alone. In my experience, and to my surprise, I've found that very few women don't want a man to join them for lunch. It's all in how you ask. Friendly. Politely. That's the key.

You can simply say, "I'm alone too, can I share your meal? I hate eating alone.

You can add with a smile, "I've been told it's very bad for digestion. Or something similar, like, "It's much nicer to eat in pleasant company."

If you walk into a restaurant and see a woman sitting alone at a counter, or if the tables are very close together (sometimes they touch, which allows the owner to seat more customers, but also creates an atmosphere that encourages people to meet and gives the restaurant a good reputation), don't hesitate and sit next to her. You can then ask her if this is her first time at the restaurant.

Whether she says yes or no, you always win. If she says no, pretend you've been there before and make a menu suggestion. This is an excellent "appetizer." If she says yes, pretend you just discovered the restaurant and ask for a suggestion. She will probably be happy that you consulted her in this way.

Speaking of restaurants, there are a few that are known for dating. Go to them. Give a generous tip. They'll remember you. And don't hesitate to tell them you want a seat next to a table where an attractive woman is sitting, either alone or with a friend. This will quickly become a convention, a kind of complicity between you and he will be happy to reserve the best tables for you. Don't forget the tip. It's Pavlov's principle. It creates a conditioned reflex in him. He will be your ally.

In restaurants, there is also a fairly common practice of offering a drink from a distance, a drink that is brought by the waiter, often accompanied by his card. This is not a bad one. However, it's a bit worn out and it's not clear if the woman who accepted your drink will want to go further. Generally, women are too polite to return the drink offered to them, but feel that this does not commit them to anything. Which, let's face it, they are absolutely right. It would be too easy.

Personally, I think a direct approach is better. At least you know where you stand. On the business card that comes with the glass, you can write a little note that can speed things up. I think a small compliment attached to a request is appropriate. The wording is up to you. You can use the inspiration of the moment. It could be something like, "Your eyes are beautiful. Would you allow me the pleasure of admiring them more closely?

Or more directly and passionately, "I wish to meet you. May I join you?"

Or the enigmatic style: "Didn't we already meet in Rome two years ago?

There is something subtly flattering about this question. If you ask her, she sounds like a woman who travels. Incidentally, you're flattering yourself. You're telling her you're a man who travels, too. Of course, you should preferably choose a city where you have already been. However, this is not mandatory. The important thing is to establish contact. After that you improvise, as we are generally all doomed to do in this world. I mentioned earlier that the glass trick is not new, but that doesn't mean it's not effective. You will probably get amazing results. Certainly, women aren't offered drinks like this every day, so this excites them. It has a romantic vibe to it. It's kind of like in the movies.

## SUPERMARKET

I'm exaggerating a bit, you might say. On the contrary, it's great. Women think of adventure everywhere, especially in a place as mundane and everyday as a supermarket. The surprise effect will be even greater. And most importantly, it can be done in a very simple and very harmless way. Moreover, the mere fact that you do your own shopping can please many women who will immediately think that you are not a macho, that you believe in equality of the two sexes since you do not despise such a domestic task. There are many opportunities to approach a woman in a supermarket. At the vegetable counter, you can ask her, for example, where the hell they put the watercress, which is nowhere to be found. Or you can ask for advice on what product to buy. If she's trying to reach an item on the top shelf and its size makes it hard to do, you rush to help. At the checkout line, you might complain about the wait time. One thing is for sure, don't neglect supermarkets. You'll see, you'll have your work cut out for you....

## STORES

The stores are golden places. There are not only customers, but also saleswomen, many of whom are very pretty. The advantage with them is that they are obligated to answer you.

Personally, I've made three delightful conquests with salespeople. And do you know why? Or rather how? Simply by being nice to them. Most customers are in a hurry, impatient and rather dry with salesgirls. If you are courteous, chat with her, make a few jokes, she will be pleased. Your presence is refreshing. You are a change from the old men who nag her all day.

Don't hesitate to ask her opinion. She will be flattered. You can ask her to advise you on buying a gift for your sister or your mother, the latter being preferable, as the former may seem a little suspicious. The great thing about salespeople is that they have to talk to us and give us their time. That's the wonderful thing about them.

Another department that is excellent is the men's clothing department. Pick out clothes for yourself and ask the saleswoman for suggestions. Ask her what looks good on you. Tell her that you really appreciate a female opinion. With female customers, you can use a similar tactic. If the saleswoman is not nearby and a beautiful woman is near you, don't hesitate to ask her opinion. Last year I met an exquisite woman who was using this technique. I simply asked her in the simplest way possible, "Sorry to bother you, Miss, but I have a big problem, maybe you can help me?" (There is something reassuring about asking for a favor.

This is something that few women will dare refuse you unless they are totally uncivilized. This has the advantage of not committing to anything. The woman doesn't feel affected. Even if she has it and is happy, it doesn't make her feel bad. A crucial detail with many women). Well, I'll take care of that. Maybe you could help me," I said. I can't decide between this tie or that tie, this shirt or that shirt.... (optional of course).

I won't tell you the rest. You wouldn't believe me. You'll think I'm trying to portray myself as an irresistible seducer. In fact, this woman was shopping because she was bored. She was feeling sad. She was subconsciously searching for the soul who would comfort her. You can be sure there are countless women like her.

## Museums

Many women visit museums, especially in the afternoon, for the same reasons. They are bored. Of course, there are real art lovers. But even they can get bored. The best thing to do is to simply stop in front of a painting that the woman is looking at and leave a comment. There are several types. It can be, "I don't understand how Gauguin could become famous with such paintings. "

If she is a Gauguin specialist, you can be sure she will respond. A discussion will probably follow. As for the rest, there's no need to draw a picture for you, is there? You've broken the ice, that's what matters. You can also ask, in a more neutral way, "What do you think of this painting? Or, "What period is this painting from, say, Picasso?

Of course, if she is totally ignorant, you might embarrass her. But then she might think you know a little bit about it, if you can ask these questions, and you might interest her. You can also say, "I don't understand anything about this painting. What do you think the painter was trying to get at?"

He probably won't understand what you're getting at right away. You'll build his confidence. Go for small, successive touches. Play the pointillist... It's obvious that the encounters you'll have in a museum will be of a different kind than those you might have on the street. So it depends on the type of women you're looking for.

## COURSES AND SCHOOLS

I won't go into too much detail about the schools. I gave you an example earlier where I won over a classmate in my German classes. Women feel safe in such an environment and because there is a common interest, it makes things much easier. In the group discussions that often take place in class, it's easy to get noticed by the woman you're interested in.

After class, you can go up to her and tell her you would like her to explain why she thinks this or that, or what she thinks about a theory the teacher just presented. There are endless courses you can take.

Obviously I would recommend the ones where men are outnumbered. Auto mechanics classes can be exciting, but they are almost never attended by women. On the other hand, dance classes, gymnastics classes, cooking classes, even, will probably put you in the minority. This is probably one of the few times when it's good to be. Enjoy. Women can take the first steps on their own. A rivalry may develop over you. Women will want to know which of them will be the first to attract your interest. You will be the sole beneficiary.

## THE BEACH

At the beach, especially on vacation, there are countless opportunities. The sun, the sea, the salt air, the laziness, the distance from the usual scenery, all contribute to the taste of adventure. It's almost too easy.

If you spot a girl, you lie down next to her. You can ask her for a light, offer her a cigarette. The possibilities are endless. If all the places around her are occupied, you can accidentally throw a balloon at her, then apologize but start a conversation. If it's very hot, as it often is, you can offer her a drink while you have one.

## PARKS

Parks are also excellent places. Many women go there to dream, read, rest. Sit on the same bench. These are public benches, you need to remember that. If she's reading, ask her if it's interesting. If you happen to have already read it, you can of course discuss it.

## CLUBS, DISCOS

It is obviously the most natural place to pick up a woman. At least the one that men spontaneously think of when they want to meet someone. If you don't already know, most women go there for the same reason you do. Of course, there may be some purists who go just for the dancing. But that's the small number.

It is primarily a meeting place. There are countless techniques to use. We'll talk about them in the next chapter. I just want to say one thing. Do you want to know who I think is the easiest woman to pick up? I guess so, since you're reading this book. Well, it's the woman who goes to a club by herself.

Despite the feminist revolution, there is still a strong prejudice against women going out without a date or at least without a girlfriend. There are also many places where a woman alone is not allowed.

So for a woman to face prejudice and dare to go to a bar or club by herself, she must really want to meet someone. Almost desperately so. If you find yourself in the same situation, don't hesitate to approach her. You can share your loneliness. So be on the lookout. If you spot a lonely woman in a bar, there's a nine out of ten chance she'll be happy to talk to you. I'm not saying she'll necessarily like you, I'm not saying she'll jump into your arms and be in her bed that night, but she won't reject you. That's already a good point for you.

## EVERYWHERE...

Of course, it would be useless to try to make an exhaustive list of places where you can meet people, make contact, since we said at the beginning that you can "pick up" anywhere. So don't hesitate. And take advantage of every opportunity.

# 5. THE FIRST CONTACT

As we move into this new chapter, you need to know something very simple but something that some men have never stopped to think about. What it takes to seduce a woman is simply to talk to her. Yes, it is that simple. I can also tell you that if you can talk to women, make verbal contact with them, you will undoubtedly succeed in seducing many of them.

What prevents men from talking to women, from trying to get to know them, is usually the fear of rejection. Of course, not all women will say yes. But you'll be surprised at how many women won't say no, or at least won't reject you, because you talked to them, and they'll be glad you did.

Remember this: simply having the courage to approach a woman makes her feel good about you. Most men don't dare do that. So you walk away with an advantage. It shows that you don't care about rigid social conventions, that you know how to dare. Women like that. And don't forget that women are often as embarrassed as you are about being tried.

You will find that with practice you will develop confidence. It is usually the beginning that is difficult, in any field. After a while, approaching a woman will be the most natural thing in the world for you. You will make mistakes. You'll be rejected. But that's okay. As they say, one lost, ten found. And after all, nothing is ever lost. It's an extra experience.

It's perfectly fine to talk to women, you might say, but you still need to know what to say to them. I want to emphasize from the outset that what you tell them in the beginning is relatively secondary. What matters is simply breaking the ice, making the first contact. You don't need to have the wit of Voltaire or Sacha Guitry. Originality is not even necessary, even if you can show it, it can also be effective. In this field, the most trivial tricks, the most trivial recipes can be wonderfully successful.

You can simply ask a woman, very casually, "Haven't we met somewhere before? "

Or a variation, "I think we know each other, don't we? "

Or, "Do you live in the 6th or Saint-Germain? (Preferably choose a neighborhood or, if applicable, a nice city).

"Did you study at the Collège Henri IV? "It's trivial, isn't it? I warned you.

But it's also usually very effective. And that's what counts. After all, anglers have been using the same lures for centuries, and that doesn't make the fish hard. One of the advantages of these starters is more subtle than it sounds. All of these questions are really flattering. They imply that you think you recognize the person. If you remember their face, then there is something remarkable about them. No one likes to go unnoticed. When you feel differently, you are almost always flattered.

Here are a few staples you can use depending on your circumstances.

Are you by any chance Gemini? (Or any other sign, with a reservation for Virgo, unless you want to create an effect whose outcome I can't predict). You may or may not like it. It depends. Some women will find it a bit of a pain in the ass. I think if the woman is very young, it's still acceptable. If not, wait until you are further along in the conversation.

*Hi. Good evening.*

This is probably the simplest. The disadvantage is that it is not a question and does not lead to an answer. The woman can always return your greeting and things can stay as they are. This is what you want to avoid above all else. Remember this. In general, it is best to ask a question. The woman can then return the favor. This makes things easier for her. Remember that she is also intimidated by being approached by a stranger. In this regard, remember that approaching a woman is still, in some ways, also very sophisticated, a kind of aggression, even if the intention is good. After all, you are a stranger. Politeness and kindness are generally the best way to go, although a more chivalrous approach can sometimes have excellent results.

*Do you know where I can find a similar book?*

Or is it a good novel? (In a bookstore or library, anywhere you meet a woman with a book in her hand).

*What color are your eyes?*

They are absolutely beautiful. (In general, women really appreciate compliments regarding their eyes).

*Your name is not Suzanne by any chance? Are you a dancer?*

This is very flattering. Girls, thousands of women have dreamed of one day becoming a ballerina. By asking her this question, you are implicitly telling her that you think she is stylish and fashionable.

Equally excellent variation: are you a model or an actress?

It's one of my favorites. Even more women have dreamed or dream of becoming an actress someday. Since actresses are generally very beautiful, it's always a treat. And it usually makes for an easy follow-up. If she's an actress (odds are slim), well, that's wonderful! She'll think you recognized her. If she's not, she might say she was part of an amateur theater group, or that she did some shots for a photographer friend, or maybe even a commercial.

A variation: *You look like Isabelle Adjani or Catherine Deneuve, are you related to her by any chance?*

Of course, there is no family connection. But the resemblance is flattering. Very flattering. Of course, the similarity has to be plausible. I once used a similar introduction. I was in a club when I saw a beautiful woman. Brown hair, blue eyes, bright teeth, full lips.

Just my type. In fact, most men's type, at least judging by the vultures that hovered around her but didn't dare speak to her. Vultures, that's a good comparison. Most men are like vultures with women: they wait for something to happen, for her to die, so to speak, before swooping down on her.

That's the mistake. A mistake that doesn't make me laugh. I desperately wanted to talk to this woman. I was wondering what I was going to say to her when I noticed her great resemblance to Gala, the woman who had been the painter Dali's partner for years. I approached her as she was dancing and said, "I have to tell you. I've been watching you dance for a while now and I just found out who you look like: Gala, Dali's wife.

She smiled. By a strange coincidence, she was a painter. You're going to tell me I'm lucky. Yes, you are. But the game wasn't won yet. In fact, it was rather long. I had to insist on getting her phone number. But I was able to get a first meeting. Nothing happened on the first date. The second one was a pleasant surprise. She invited me to her house. Then, after an hour, he told me point blank, "Take off your shirt, I want to see what you look like.

Pretty cool, huh? I'll spare you the rest because we need to get back to the serious stuff.

*Are you Swedish, German, Swiss?*

Maybe you've never met a Swiss woman, or a Swedish or German, who don't necessarily look special, but are usually flattering. But you should avoid some nationalities, as the prejudice against them can be very strong. Use your own judgment. And if it's a black woman with brown eyes, don't ask her if she's Swedish.

*What kind of dog is it?*

In a park. Or on the street. If you have a dog too, that's even better.

*You look sad, is something wrong?*

I've never used it. There's nothing stopping you from doing it if you feel like it. I prefer its corollary:

What makes you look so happy? I'd like to meet you.

*You have a very nice hat.*

*I would love to meet you.*

*Are you alone?* She nods. *So am I. Shall we have a chat?*

One of my best. Simple. Friendly. Easy for everyone to do. And it doesn't compromise you. Sometimes it's okay not to find out your game right away. Misunderstanding has surprising virtues. Also, because it is purely friendly, the woman feels more secure.

*Excuse me, miss. May I ask you the name of your dentist?*

He has really impressive teeth and he shows them off. Listen: he smiles a lot.

*Haven't I met you before in London, in Venice?* You seem to be a great traveler before the Lord. Your question implies that you also travel. This is a good thing.

*What can you drink?*

At a bar. If he has a glass of beer, don't. If his drink looks special, then it is excellent. She will probably be happy to show the originality of her taste. We will see later that one of the best ways to seduce a woman is to allow her to show her taste. Everything you do or say should reflect an advantageous image of herself.

*Can I buy you a drink?*

Simple. But it has proven itself. To be recommended.

*Do you have a light? Do you want a cigarette?* Obviously very trivial. But if you feel that the woman has already noticed you, it does not matter. She will be happy that you approached her. Remember the initial remarks I made. What you say is no big deal. The important thing is to take the first step, break the ice.

*Do you want to sit down?*

In a crowded bistro, a bar, a nightclub. It's a gallantry that's always in order. It doesn't compromise you. You present yourself as a gentleman. Women like that.

Can I give you a ride somewhere? You're in your car and you see a beautiful woman waiting for the bus or looking for a cab. This technique requires a little more daring, I agree. But you'd be surprised at how many women are willing to get into a stranger's car. My former boss was a fan of this technique. He was a Swiss man in his 50s, not an Apollo. But he had a lot of spunk and verve. A true gentleman. He called this technique from an American expression, a "pick-up." Some days he felt a little sad and would take his car on the streets of Paris in the early afternoon, just after lunchtime. On the afternoons when he didn't return to the office, I knew, because he'd made me aware, that he'd hit the jackpot. The next day he would tell me about his adventure.

I was always surprised by the number of women he had in the car. Because at least one out of every two women who agreed to come in, also agreed to have a drink. My boss's hobby was champagne. Dom Pérignon. So, more often than not, the adventure ended in the afternoon to his complete satisfaction. If you don't believe me, try your luck, you'll be surprised at the result. As for beautiful women hitchhiking, don't hesitate to catch them. They are generally not shy about it. However, you don't have to try to seduce her right away. You can simply ask for her phone number. Since you have obliged her by driving her home, she will rarely dare to refuse you her phone number.

*Do you know where the post office is?*

*What is a funny box in...?* (a city where you don't live).

This is excellent. You look like a tourist. A little lost. Maybe the woman will agree to be your guide.

*You have a very pretty smile.*

This is less embarrassing than telling a woman, "You're beautiful. But it's probably just as effective.

*Can I take your picture?*

You're walking down the street with your camera (it doesn't have to be a Nikon) and you see a woman you like. You tell her that you were struck by her beauty, or the originality of her face, that you're convinced she must be insanely photogenic, and you offer her a little impromptu photo session.

In general, most women accept. For one simple reason. It's extremely flattering. And it doesn't commit you to anything. You can add to reassure her that you're an amateur photographer and that you plan to enter a contest. Or that you're taking photography classes with the goal of becoming a professional. If she refuses, saying that she's in a hurry, that she doesn't have time, offer to meet her at another time.

Ask for her phone number and explain that you've never seen a face as expressive or special as hers. Success is almost guaranteed. If she agrees to an immediate photo session, you should get her phone number so you can give her the photos when they are developed. If the session has gone on for, say, ten minutes (take your time), you can then buy her a drink to thank her for her kindness.

In the conversation that happens before or during, don't ask the woman if she's a model or actress or if she's done at least a few pictures in a magazine. All points in your favor for the reason I explained earlier. This technique is one of the best. You will be surprised how many foreign women will agree to come to your home for a photo shoot.

*Do you want to make love?*

To be blunt, you can hardly be more blunt. Forgive the brutality of this introduction. But I couldn't finish my list without mentioning this question, which, while not lacking in boldness, still arises. It depends for whom and with whom. I have to tell you, I haven't tried it often.

Only once, in fact. But it was positive. Let me tell you about it. I arrived at a club one weekday evening. I was groggy and needed some company. When I arrived, I saw a girl dancing by herself. She wasn't extraordinarily beautiful. But she was extremely sensual, with a rather generous chest. Maybe she would be just as generous with herself with me. At least that's what I was hoping for. She had to be at least thirty years old. This is a very important detail.

Women of this age have seen the rain. They are less likely to be frightened. Also, the sexuality of women in their 30s is generally much more satisfied and vibrant than that of younger women. They have more brutal, stronger desires that are more like our own. If the woman I was about to approach had only been eighteen, I probably would have refrained or simply refused.

After a few minutes of reflection (if you can call the desires and images running through my mind reflection), I decided to go straight there. I walked to the dance floor and approached her. I hesitated. I danced for a few moments to give myself a few more seconds of "reflection".

I almost gave up. He would tell me to get lost. Or he would slap me. I finally went.

Can I ask you a direct question? - Yes," she said, slightly surprised.

- Do you want to make love?

She didn't answer yes. But she didn't answer no. Instead, she said:

- Perhaps we could discuss this.

I was delighted and amazed, in a way. We sat down. I offered him a drink. We got to know each other. In the brief moments of silence that punctuated our conversation, I told myself that eventually this woman (whose name, incidentally, was Helene) would not be able to answer my question in the affirmative. She didn't know me. She didn't know my name. How could she follow a stranger who could be a dangerous maniac? After two hours of conversation, I had to negotiate. I wanted to invite her to my home for coffee. At first she declined, saying she had to get up early the next day, which didn't seem like a good excuse.

"We'll have a little coffee," I said, "and I'll drive you home right after.

He eventually agreed. My insistence was soon rewarded. Half an hour later, to my amazement, even though we barely knew each other, he was screaming that he loved me. Now that's modernism! I must confess, however, that this wonderfully voluptuous adventure had regrettable consequences. In fact, by temporarily curing my lovesickness, Hélène had given me the so-called lovesickness. What do you want? When a woman agrees to follow you home on the first night, chances are you're not the first to whom she does these spontaneous favors. Nor the last.

He may have followed a stranger the day before under similar circumstances....

*The "love letter".*

A very interesting method - especially for shy people - is to write a love letter to a stranger and keep it with you at all times.

As soon as you see an attractive woman, you hand her the letter. Of course, it is necessary that this letter is handwritten, on beautiful paper, and that you have several letters with you. The formula is mathematical: the more letters you deliver, the greater your chances of success. You can hand over the letter and say, "This letter is for you, read it later," or even keep quiet and blush!

What should we remember from all this? There are many effective ways to approach a woman. There are dozens that you can point to or have probably already used. It's almost limitless. Like I said before, don't be afraid of the trivial. The ends justify the means. The old stuff usually works. If they didn't, they'd never become old stuff. But don't be afraid to be spontaneous, to be inspired by the moment, to be original. With some reservations, however. Because of course, if the sight of a stranger inspires thoughts of a sado-masochistic nature in you, it's probably best to censor yourself, at least temporarily.

Before we close this chapter, let me make one final point. Despite practice, you will not succeed with all women. Did you know that a seducer like Warren Beattie, who has been called Mr. Hollywood, who has seduced beautiful women like Julie Christie, Diane Keaton, Joan Collins, and who is rumored to have had an affair with the beautiful Isabelle Adjani, even though he was twenty years older than her, did you know that he admitted to being successful with women only once out of two times? Don't forget that he is extremely handsome, wealthy and famous and his reputation as a knight precedes him wherever he goes.

Paradoxically, women are often only attracted to a man's reputation as a ladies' man. What's liked will be liked, you might say. So you, who are neither rich nor famous and probably do not have the physique of this American actor, it is normal that a number of women reject your advances. Most likely more than one time out of two. My experience has taught me that one success in seven or eight attempts is a very respectable average. An average that you can easily reach and that, contrary to what you might think, will not improve much with time.

One in seven women isn't much, you might say. That means I'll have to take six rejections. That's not good. It's not serious at all. It's not the death of a man. And it means this: if you meet a woman every day, the law of averages being what it is, you'll be able to get one woman a week if you feel like it.

# 6. WHAT DO WE SAY NEXT?

In his million-copy book, How to Win Friends, Dale Carnegie outlines six ways to win people's sympathy. I'll quote them verbatim.

- Rule 1. Show genuine interest in others.

- Rule 2. Smile.

- Rule 3. Remember that a man's name is the sweetest and most important word in his vocabulary.

- Rule 4. Be a good listener. Encourage others to speak up for themselves.

- Rule 5. Talk to the person you're talking to about what they like.

- Rule 6. Make him feel genuinely important.

These rules apply to both women and men. But what should you do once you've made initial contact with a woman? You simply have to win her over.

This is what flirting is all about. Winning a woman's sympathy. Reread the six rules Dale Carnegie laid out. (I highly recommend you read his book.) These rules are deeper than you might think at first glance. Also, as paradoxical as it may seem, if you want to know what a woman likes, observe yourself, ask yourself what you like.

Who are the people around you who have won your sympathy? Is it the ones who only talk about themselves, who never care about you, never smile, never listen when you talk and make you feel like a minus habens? Of course not. These are the others. Perhaps they are rarer. But beings who apply these principles with those around them quickly become incredibly popular. People are drawn to them like a magnet. The basic functioning of women is very similar to that of men.

# THE MAGIC OF DESIRE

It can be said in a general way, that is, without taking into account the inevitable exceptions, that it is not necessarily the most handsome men who are most successful with women, but those who love them the most, those who desire them the most. Women love to be desired, to be loved, much more than to be reduced, for example, to contemplating a handsome man who is not really interested in them. For my part, I can say without any pretense, as a simple and almost clinical observation on the effects of desire, that I have almost always succeeded in seducing the women I really wanted. Fiercely. Violently, without showing it, of course.

On the other hand, I've had a much higher number of failures with women who inspired only lukewarm desire. Everything happens as if the woman's desire responds exactly to what you project toward her. This is probably the equivalent of the law of causality. Action equals reaction. For my part, I decided to only go after women I really liked. Honestly. My desire is stronger. The compliments I give her are more sincere. So more convincing. My eloquence is more natural.

I have observed that I especially like one type of woman who, by a coincidence that is probably not a coincidence, is my type. I have little success with blondes. I don't mind this too much, because I've found that while I find many of them very pretty, I'm not really attracted to them, deeply. No doubt there are exceptions. But I'm speaking in general terms. You probably have a type of woman yourself. So I would suggest that if you want to increase your chances of success, you should try mostly with women you really like. This is easier and much more enjoyable.

Desire travels mysteriously as an invisible fluid. It affects women in subtle ways, on a level other than the strictly physical. Do you know what the best way to increase desire is? It's chastity. It might surprise you that I talk about chastity in a book about the art of seduction. But you'll understand. If you're a little desperate, if you're absolutely trying to meet a woman, be absolutely chaste. Don't have auto-erotic practices. Don't go see girls, I mean joy girls.

The power of your desire will radiate throughout your body and exert an occult influence on women, as it operates on an etheric level. It will give you a whole new charm and probably a state of exaltation that will make you fun and attractive. Chastity gives the eyes a special glow. The eyes have a lot to do with seduction. Try it. The strength of your controlled desire will make you bold with women. Try it. Another way to increase your sexual vitality and charm is to eat very frugally. Try it for a few days and above all be chaste. This is the best way to have adventures.

## IS SHE THE WOMAN IN YOUR LIFE?

There is an age for multiple encounters. Then comes the age when you look for the love of your life. For those who are dissatisfied with their love life, who regularly seduce women, but would like to meet the woman of their life, observe the same rule.

Be Chaste. Don't accept mediocrity and compromise. Tell yourself that you will never touch a woman again until you meet the woman you really like, the soulmate you are looking for. In my opinion, this is the best way to get to know her. Quickly. Without you having to do anything special to meet her. Don't go out more than usual. She will come to you, mysteriously attracted by the purity of your desire and its power.

To quickly find the woman in your life, be chaste until you meet her. Believe me. Life is more mysterious than you think. And so are the laws of love.

## IT IS UNIQUE...

What repels most women is the feeling that a man is trying to seduce her just because she's a woman, that if it's not her, it will be someone else, that he's not really interested in her. You need to make her feel that she is unique, that she is special, that you really find her interesting. Do you know what is the surest way to make her feel unique?

It's getting serious. I'm going to give you a very simple way that has wonderful results. Tell yourself. In fact, all people are exciting, unique, fascinating. But unfortunately, we don't realize it. We are obsessed with our little selves. We don't see the people around us. We live in a kind of sleep that we don't even know about. In my opinion, this is the great tragedy of people. They never see each other. They don't really communicate. Why is that? The reason I'm about to give you will probably surprise you, but it's the real reason.

People don't see themselves, aren't fascinated by their peers and life in general simply because they lack focus. Yes, they lack concentration. Their mind is dissipated. Their view of reality and beings is constantly distracted by all the thoughts running through their minds. They are not living in the moment. Hic et nunc.

I'm going to give you a very simple little exercise that I can tell will transform your life. Please practice it regularly.

Focus is the real key to happiness. You can finally live in the present, without worrying about the past or the future. This even leads to a kind of ecstasy. The exercise is simple. You may have heard of it.

Draw a black dot on a wall or the floor. Sit comfortably (this can be a yoga position such as lotus or Samaritan) and stare at the dot. Don't blink. Keep your eyelids open. This is very important. You may find it difficult at first. You may feel a tingling in your eyes. Don't worry about this. This exercise strengthens the optic nerve and can also help correct some vision defects. Constant practice of this exercise will give your eyes a magnetic appeal, they will shine with a new radiance.

At first, do it for a few minutes. Then you can increase to half an hour or more. Personally, I keep doing it until I have tears running down my cheeks. And believe me, I have excellent eyesight despite my incessant intellectual work. The steady gaze is very important. It will calm your thoughts and make them clearer. This seemingly simple exercise has extraordinary effects. As surprising as it may seem, it will help you understand your destiny. You will have this very strong feeling. You will have totally new thoughts. You will see who you are. You will say to yourself: this is me. Words are obviously inadequate to describe this very special feeling.

You will also feel this way about those around you. You will no longer see people in the same way.

way. In fact, you'll really feel like you're seeing them for the first time. You'll be fascinated by people and moved. Your prejudices will fall away. You'll love people in a new way. You will feel their drama. You will be attentive to who they are. The more you are able to pay attention to the little black dot on the floor or wall, the more you will be able to pay attention to others. This attention you'll see has an extraordinary effect on people. They will be irresistibly drawn to you. Enthused.

If you want to get the most out of this little concentration exercise, I recommend accompanying it with a focus on your breath. Take a deep breath. Most importantly, exhale completely. The key to breathing is in the exhale. If you want even faster and more amazing results, accompany this exercise with the repetition of a mantra. A mantra is a sacred word with a magical effect. I won't go into detail on this subject. There are whole books on the subject. And I emphasize that you don't have to believe in mantras to feel their effects. I will give you two mantras that are very powerful and come from two very ancient traditions. The first one is the Hu mantra (pronounced I-or). You have to separate it into two. First you pronounce I and then you extend the Ou. It is a very soft sound that calms the mind and makes it easier to concentrate. It will also give you other benefits that I won't talk about here, but you can find out for yourself. The second mantra I give you is longer. It is the following: OM NAMA SHIVAYA. It means: I bow to Shiva, who is a deity in the East. I suggest you mentally repeat it while looking at the black spot.

There is another way to do the concentration exercise. It is the frontal gaze. Always keeping your eyes open, without blinking them, fix the point between the two eyebrows, at the root of the nose, where resides what occultists call the third eye. This is the seat of intelligence.

This exercise has an amazing effect. It will make your intelligence

extremely lively and untied. It will also open up a new universe for you, which I will leave to you. You also practice it by repeating one or the other of the mantras. Start with a few minutes. At first, your eyes will tire quickly. Keep at it. Something surprising awaits you at the end of the road. Faster than you think. Try to do two sessions a day, one in the morning and one in the evening. You can also do these exercises with your eyes closed and focus on your third eye. It depends on your disposition. Choose the way that works best for you.

Regular practice of these exercises will transform your life after a few months. Your face will be bathed in a new light. You will exert a magnetic charm on people, both men and women. Practice. Focus. Repeat the mantra. Meditate. Happiness is within your grasp. And success.

## THE ART OF PLEASURE

I don't know if you've noticed, but the art of pleasing is essentially in the art of talking. Women," said actress Madeleine Renaud, "are like rabbits, you grab them by the ears.

Nothing could be further from the truth. And probably the most touching thing for a woman when a man speaks is compliments. Don't hesitate to give them. Intelligently. In an original way. For example, if a woman is known to have beautiful eyes, chances are that a hundred men before you have told her so. She won't mind, of course, because we rarely tire of compliments, but you'll impress her more if you explain why her eyes are beautiful. Or discover a more subtle, less obvious beauty in her. Maybe she has beautiful eyebrows, or exquisite cheekbones. Or very well-defined lips. This will please her much more. If you don't hesitate to be a little Machiavellian and you've noticed that her nose isn't perfect, simply tell her that you think it's cute. She probably has a complex about it. She will be absolutely delighted. In general, don't forget that a woman's physical appearance is one of her constant concerns. Vanity is her Achilles heel. If you want to get your kicks, attack that heel....

As soon as you know his name, don't hesitate to say it, often. It is sweet music to his ears. It is a kind of compliment.

If you have a sense of humor, don't hesitate to use it. Make her laugh. Half of all women fall in love with a man who makes them laugh. Personally, it's a rule for me to say anything. Literally anything that comes to mind. Women love it. It balances laughter and seriousness. This is the ideal. Otherwise, the woman may not take you seriously. And smile. The effect of a smile is incredible. A smile brightens the face. It is the sign of success and happiness. Don't be stingy with it. It is the key to many hearts.

## WHAT TO TALK ABOUT?

About everything and nothing. About the rain and the sun. If you're passionate about running, German literature, travel, Truffaut movies, talk about it. A passionate person is often passionate. Enthusiasm is contagious. Nothing is more boring for a woman than a man who seems to be interested in nothing. However, by all means, avoid bragging. It's only enjoyable for you.

## BEING A GOOD LISTENER

Talking is important, but listening is much more important. And, certainly, it is much rarer. The self-centeredness of most people is astounding. How many times have we witnessed conversations that were just two sad monologues, each person rushing to tell the other what he or she wanted to say, without really listening.

If you regularly practice the small concentration exercises I've explained, this is a problem you won't encounter. You will be fascinated by people. You will listen to them attentively. With real pleasure. With real fascination. You will be interested in what the woman you want to seduce says. Get her to talk. About her. About what she is interested in. What she's passionate about. I've experienced this many times. Getting the other person to talk about themselves is the greatest pleasure you can give them. It's a form of compliment. It's saying, I'm interested in you, I'm passionate about you.

Women often fear that they are only interested in and enjoy their physical qualities. By getting her to talk about herself, it reassures her. It shows her that the man is interested in her personality. Of course, this does not mean that you should not tell her that you find her beautiful.

I was often told by a woman at the end of an hour-long conversation that she enjoyed talking to me. But I had hardly talked at all. I had only been listening. And she asked a few questions to get her going again. We had talked about her. She was overjoyed.

That being said, men are equal to women in this regard. When listening to a woman, don't be afraid to look her in the eye. Stare. Without blinking. This has a profound effect. It confirms her feeling that you are really interested in her. There is nothing more irritating than talking to someone who is constantly looking away. Most people are intoxicated by their little selves. Their drug is their person. Unfortunately, human beings are selfish monsters who stubbornly refuse to think only of your pleasure....

"There is only one bad genre," Voltaire said of literature, "the boring genre." The same can be said of conversation. Above all, avoid serious, formal conversations. Women don't like them. Also avoid talking about the countless problems you have, the problems you have at work, the nervous breakdown you feel on the horizon. Women prefer to have fun, to laugh, at least during a first meeting.

One medicine that can be successful, though I prescribe it with some reservation (it's a matter of tact and convenience), is to talk about erotic topics. Elegantly. (Especially avoid vulgarity. It can only appeal to certain women. This is the exception). You'll be surprised, however, at how many women fall for this little game and talk about very intimate topics. It's all about the right balance. It's about knowing how to assess the woman in front of you.

I don't think it's necessary to address these issues directly. You can eroticize a woman more safely, or at least just as effectively, simply by making her laugh or giving her compliments. Also, if your desire for her is strong, she will feel it without you having to put it into words.

One thing I strongly recommend, however, is that you touch her, not just with your words, but physically. This creates warmth, intimacy. Needless to say, you should limit yourself (until further notice) to certain body parts. For me, my favorite part is my forearm. Which I embrace. Just for a moment. Don't let your hand linger too long. More than a few seconds and the woman will likely be embarrassed. It becomes a sign of ownership.

You can also touch her hand, her shoulder. Toss gently if she just made you laugh or said something nice. Even the cheek. If she has nice hair and you tell her so, you can accompany your words with a gesture. You can then add that it is very silky or has an odd texture. Your gesture should not feel like a caress. It is not a sexual gesture but a friendly, warm gesture. In no way should it feel like aggression. But don't make too many of these gestures. When you touch a woman, she will feel safer and find you warmer.

## How to conclude?

The end of the night is coming. What to do? How do you end a meeting? Here more than anywhere else, you need to be psychological. Should you openly ask to spend the night with her? Or simply offer to drive her home? Should you invite her to your home for coffee? Or simply ask for her phone number? Or make an appointment? I can only make suggestions. And it's very optional. It all depends on what you want from this woman. If you are very much in love with her and you are afraid of losing her, it is better that you just ask for her phone number. You will see her again and she will advise you in due time. You should not rush things.

If you are dying to have sex with the woman you spent the evening with, you can simply tell her, for example, "I desire you so much and find you extremely sensual. Why don't we spend the night together? I'm sure it will be great."

When in doubt, always offer to walk the woman home. A good way to make the big proposal without actually doing it is to try kissing her on the doorstep. If she doesn't push you away, if she is cooperative or better yet, gets passionate, then don't hesitate. Even pretend that it's already understood that you're about to make love. Say for example, "Come on, let's go to your house.

If your kisses and caresses were fiery enough, there should be no problem. If she still refuses, don't get upset. She may not want to be seen as a novice girl, even though she wants sex as much as you do. You could try pushing a little. But not too much. You'll probably be successful with her on the second night anyway.

In general, on the first evening, I observed that, if anything, they had an apartment, women preferred to go to their homes, especially if they had only known us for a few hours. This is normal. They feel more secure. You have to give in to this preference, which I find exquisite. Discovering a woman's bedroom always seemed very erotic to me.

There is a clue that can guide you to end the evening, to know what to do and how far to go, to use Cocteau's famous expression. Think about the evening you just had and especially the quality of the contact you had with the woman. It has often happened to me to talk so passionately with some women, to have such a beautiful exchange that, strictly speaking, and without our realizing it, we were already making love.

In these situations, I don't hesitate to be quite direct.

"Let's spend the night together?" is a good formula that has brought me success. A romantic variation: "It was such an interesting evening, it's a shame we have to part. Why don't we spend the night together?

You can add, "Even if we don't make love. I just want to be with you. I still have so much to tell you."

Well, that's up to you. However, if you got a phone number or an appointment, it's a success. It will soon become a reality.

# 7. ADVICE, THOUGHTS, STRATEGY ISSUES....

Is it better to go out alone, with a partner or in a group? This is a very important question. Personally, I strongly advise against gang dating.

It's vulgar and women won't take you seriously. Your chances of success are limited. Two is much better. This has undeniable advantages for the simple reason that women go out more often with a friend than alone, especially in clubs and discos.

Since the law of probability is that you and your boyfriend rarely like both women, agree in advance so that one of you makes concessions. Take turns. There's a variation of double dating that I think is a superior form. At least in terms of effectiveness. Instead of going with a boyfriend, go with a girlfriend. You'll be surprised at the results. You agree in advance to give each other complete latitude. Rivalry between women plays an important role in the attractiveness of a man. Paradoxically, a man who is accompanied is almost always more interesting to women. Especially if he seems to be available despite everything. Many women like to steal a man from another woman. It is a test of their charm.

There is still the option of going out on your own. For me, this is the one I prefer. It's the simplest. It gives you the most freedom of movement. You don't have to discuss with your boyfriend whether or not he wants to go after a particular woman. Also, you can approach both a single woman and two women together.

When you approach two women together, it gives you a great advantage to be alone. At least if you know how to maneuver. Since it's very rare for two very beautiful women to date (I don't know why, maybe it's beyond their strengths), there's usually one you're more interested in.

I'm going to give you some advice that I think is very helpful. The first is to not focus exclusively on the interesting woman. There are several reasons for this.

The first is that it would be a lack of basic politeness. You always have to look like a gentleman. Also, they are both engaged, you would probably embarrass the interesting woman by neglecting to take an interest in her friend.

But the most subtle benefit of this strategy is that it leaves doubt in the mind of the woman you've chosen. This puts you in a position of strength. Despite the likely friendship between the two women, a certain rivalry arises between them. A rivalry that is to your advantage. Of course, don't prolong the suspense indefinitely. This could be detrimental to you.

## WOMEN SIGNALS

In any exchange between two people, the interlocutors emit signals. Club meetings are obviously no exception. Reading these often subtle signals can be a great help in dating. Despite women's pseudo-liberation, they generally remain less resourceful than men. They generally leave the first steps to men. However, they generally give signals to indicate their interest. They have attitudes and gestures.

I have observed that often an interested woman, even if she does not dare to approach you directly, will be able to subtly approach you to get you to talk to her. In this regard, I made another observation. If you notice that a woman has just made such an approach, don't wait too long to respond. It took a lot of courage for her to dare such an approach. If you wait more than ten minutes, her vanity will be hurt. She will convince herself that you are not interested and leave. The best thing to do is to talk to her within a few minutes of her arrival. Why not immediately? This will charm her. She will congratulate herself for taking the opportunity. This will show her that she did not go unnoticed, that you noticed her immediately.

There are of course more obvious signs, the easiest to decipher is the gaze, repetitive or insistent. If a woman regularly looks in your direction, it means that she has noticed you and probably likes you. So don't hesitate, approach her. You will almost certainly be successful.

If a woman asks you for a light or a cigarette, chances are it's an apology. She is interested in you. If she approaches you herself, if she asks if you've met before, that's usually wonderful. These are clear signs of her interest.

If the woman smiles at you from afar, this is another extremely favorable sign. Do not hesitate to walk towards her. She finds you sympathetic.

Once you have approached her, the woman continues to give off signals that speak volumes. If she uses the same techniques with you that I have been trying to communicate to you, all will be well. If, for example, she compliments you on your outfit, if she thinks you look like a comedian, if she tells you that you're nice and that she likes talking to you, that you're funny, you're on the right track.

There are also nonverbal signals. He laughs out loud at your every joke, he smiles all the time, he touches you. These are all positive signs. Observe his body position. If he sways his body imperceptibly in your direction, if he tends to move closer to you, a closer approach may be possible.

## YOU REAP WHAT YOU SOW

I would be remiss if I didn't finish this little book without a word of warning. Flirting is wonderful. It allows you to make new contacts, to make girlfriends and lovers. But you must not forget this: you must be careful and fair. Many women are very sensitive, very vulnerable. It's easy to hurt them by making promises that you don't keep. I recommend basic honesty. Be honest. Lay your cards on the table. Don't promise love when all you're looking for is pleasure. Don't put yourself in situations where you would be ashamed of yourself.

He who has caused pain will suffer. I have experienced this to my cost and it is only fair. There always comes a time when, in a righteous way, we are accountable. Life takes the most unbelievable turns to put us in situations where those we have caused to suffer pay us back. Unless it's someone else.

## 8. Conclusion

Contrary to popular belief, seduction is the easiest thing in the world. As I said in the beginning, all women love to be conquered, at least if it's done with a certain elegance. Many women feel lonely and desperately want to break the cycle of their loneliness. Many women are bored in their daily lives and crave adventure.

Seduction is a very fun game that colors your life and breaks the monotony. So don't wait any longer. Dozens of interesting encounters are waiting for you, in every way. Everywhere. In the street. In the elevator. In the subway. Everywhere. We live in the century of communications. So live with your century. Communicate. Don't hesitate. It's a no-brainer. You'll be the first to be surprised by your success. Good luck!

# 9. BONUS: 101 ROMANTIC IDEAS

### IDEA # 1

If your partner is going to be gone for a few days, tell her you're worried about her and that you've hired a bodyguard.

At this point, give him a small teddy bear.

### IDEA # 2

Buy a bag of glow-in-the-dark stars and attach them to the ceiling above your bed with a message like "I love you."

When the light goes out, your message will be revealed.

### IDEA # 3

For a special occasion, buy your partner eleven real red roses and one artificial red rose. Place the artificial rose in the center of the bouquet.

Attach a note on which you wrote:

"I will love you until the last rose fades away.

### IDEA # 4

Buy your partner's domain name on the Internet, for example www.TanyaJohnston.com. Create a web page with a romantic poem and include a picture of a rose. When your partner is surfing the net, randomly ask her if she has checked if her name is being used. Have her type in the address and discover her web page.

## IDEA # 5

Buy a nice pocket mirror and gift it to your partner. Add a small card to the package that says:

"In this mirror you will see the image of the most beautiful woman in the world."

## IDEA # 6

Pick up the book your partner is reading. Using a pen, underline the letters in a chapter she hasn't read yet so you can write her a love letter.

The underlined letters will pique your partner's curiosity and hopefully she will copy your message letter by letter to decipher it. Take your time to personalize the message as much as possible, for example, "My beloved Belinda, I love you with all my heart.

## IDEA # 7

Have flowers delivered to your partner at her workplace. Not only will the flowers make her happy, but she'll also be flattered by the comments and questions from her colleagues.

## IDEA # 8

During a romantic walk, pick up a stone at the side of the path and tell your partner that you will keep this stone as a precious reminder of this happy moment.

Next, have the stone engraved with the love message of your choice and give it as a gift.

## IDEA # 9

Take a walk in the country, find a romantic hillside and lie on the grass watching the clouds.

Play, as children do, to discover shapes in the clouds.


## IDEA # 10

Get a blank sheet of paper and some colored pencils. Draw a baby picture with a smiling sun and two people holding hands. Add a bubble with your name pointing to each character and write "I love you" in a big red heart.

Then get a large envelope. Put the design in the envelope and write your partner's work address on it, making it look very official:

Send it to him in the mail so that he gets it on a day when you know your partner is busy with work.


## IDEA # 11

Memorize a Shakespeare poem and recite it to your partner when you are together in a romantic setting. Don't start reciting immediately because it may sound "prepared."

After giving her a kiss, jokingly ask her if she would like to hear you say a poem. She'll say yes, probably expecting a classic like "roses are red..."

Instead, look into her eyes and smile and recite the poem you've chosen. Her sweetly mocking smile should soon change to excitement.

## IDEA # 12

If your partner has to work late, get a tupperware and fill it with his favorite things: chocolate, herbal tea or tea, cakes.... Add his teddy bear as a bodyguard.

Stick a label on the box, "Michelle's Survival Kit," with a big red cross. Tell your partner to open the box when things get really tough.

## IDEA # 13

On an outing, get close to the children's rides and give your partner a ride.

This will remind him of the happy times of his childhood.

## IDEA # 14

Leave a rose in a place where your partner will "accidentally" find it and leave a note with a message like "Thank you for brightening my life."

## IDEA # 15

If your partner is starting a new job, buy a CD of "The Sound of Music." Record the song "I Have Confidence" on a blank CD and add your message at the end of the song. For example, you might say, "Good luck my love, I know everything will be okay. I believe in you."

Give her the CD when she leaves to listen to it on her way to work.

## IDEA # 16

Buy a small gift box, a silk square, massage oil and a business card.

Put the oil in the box after wrapping it in the silk square. Offer the package to your partner after writing, "I know a great massage therapist, good for a free trial: (Your phone number)"

## IDEA # 17

When your partner comes home from work after a particularly hard day, take a nice warm bath. Pour some scented bath oil into the tub and gently rub her from head to toe. Then take her to your room wrapped in a warm towel and have her settle into your bed with a tender kiss on her forehead.

## IDEA # 18

To do this you need a portable CD player. If you and your partner have a favorite song, make a copy of it on CD and take it with you when you go away for a romantic weekend.

When you find a romantic spot, ask your partner if they'd like to dance. Put one earbud in his ear and the second in yours and enjoy your own private dance floor.

This technique is especially effective if the location you've chosen isn't suitable for dancing, such as on top of the Empire State Building at sunset or on top of a hill during a vacation in the country.

## IDEA # 19

If your partner has a pet she loves, in addition to the gift you have planned for her, consider giving her pet a small gift as well.

## IDEA # 20

Go for a walk on the beach. Draw a big heart in the sand. Sit inside the heart and watch the sunset as you tenderly embrace your partner.

## IDEA # 21

Ask your partner to go for a walk. Take a backpack with a picnic tablecloth, crackers, cheese, some sandwiches, fruit, half a bottle of champagne and two plastic champagne flutes inside.

If your partner asks you what's in your backpack, simply say a bottle of water and two sweaters. When you've found a romantic spot, ask her if she wants to stop for a break. At this point, open your backpack and take out all the items you have inside one by one. The last item you should pull out should be the champagne.

## IDEA # 22

If you play a musical instrument, set the stage for a romantic moment where you can play for your partner.

For example, let's say you play the saxophone. Contact your friend's roommate and have your friend go out on her balcony at a specific time.

As soon as you see her appear, she starts playing a slow, romantic melody.

## IDEA # 23

You can use this idea on a day when your partner goes to work and you stay home.

Greet her on the doorstep and as soon as she leaves, email her at work. Just write, "I miss you already."

It will discover your message when it arrives at the workplace.

## IDEA # 24

If your partner has long hair, take the time to brush it slowly from roots to ends. This is especially relaxing after a shower or at bedtime.

## IDEA # 25

For a special occasion like his birthday, prepare a scavenger hunt for your partner. The game starts when you suggest a walk by the water.

When you go to the beach, take a small bag with you. The bag contains a bottle that you prepared in advance. Inside the bottle is a treasure map. To make the treasure map look real, burn the outline with a match.

While you are walking, discreetly remove the bottle from the bag and drop it in the sand at the water's edge (you may have to find a way to leave your friend behind for a few moments while you put the bottle down and retrace your steps). You will have drawn a path on the map that will lead you to a nearby bar. When you get to the coffee shop, your partner won't know what to look for; suggest that you sit down and have a coffee. When the waitress brings the coffee, she will have to suggest to your friend that what she is looking for is hidden under the slide in the children's park. And indeed, your friend will discover a key and the last piece of the treasure map. Of course, you will have worked out this scenario in advance with the waitress, who will be happy to lend a hand to a romantic man like you.

Following the directions on the map, you will arrive at the point where you have drawn a large "X" in the sand. By digging there, your partner will discover a small chest that can be opened with the key found under the slide and inside which is your gift.

## IDEA # 26

Ask your partner on a date by sending a large kraft envelope containing only a CD. On the CD, record the music from Mission Impossible, then your message that says "Your mission, if you accept, is to go to the Venoli Café, 123 Park Lane, today at 6:30 pm. There you will meet a very attractive man whom you will recognize by his red tie. The future of the free world is in your hands. This CD will self-destruct in 10 seconds. Here, record 10 beeps of a countdown and then, again, your voice saying "Damn, that didn't work! See you later..." In addition to an original invitation, you'll have made him smile.

## IDEA # 27

Contact your partner's family and ask them if there is anything your friend dreamed of when she was a child.

For example, if she has always wanted a porcelain doll, buy her one for her birthday. Not only will the gift make her happy, but the fact that you had the idea to take an interest in her desire for a child will make her happy.

## IDEA # 28

Have a portrait taken of the two of you as a couple by a professional photographer. Have the photo framed and put it on display in your home. Remember to tell your partner about this project so she has time to "look good".

### IDEA # 29

Write on a post-it note, "I think about you all day long and that makes me happy" Leave this note somewhere you are sure your partner will find it when you are gone.

### IDEA # 30

For Valentine's Day, buy your partner a pearl bracelet with at least 14 beads. Remove all the beads and have her find one bead for each of the first 14 days of February. On Valentine's Day, give her the bracelet and the remaining beads.

### IDEA # 31

When shopping at a mall, stop at a photo booth and capture this happy moment with some photos of the two of you.

Don't forget to kiss as the flash goes off.

### IDEA # 32

Leave a message on your partner's cell phone voicemail, "I just wanted to tell you that I'm thinking about you." It will always make her very happy and even more so if you hear it during a hard day at work.

### IDEA # 33

Plan a mystery trip for the two of you. Some travel agencies may offer 'surprise packages' where the destination isn't revealed until you're on the plane, or even when you arrive at your destination.

## IDEA # 34

Buy some rose petals and place them inside the sun visor on the passenger side of your car. Add a post-it note with the words "I love you" on the inside mirror of the sun visor.

During the ride, look at your partner and tell her she has something on her cheek. When she tilts the sun visor to look at herself in the rearview mirror, she'll receive a shower of rose petals and discover your little note.

## IDEA # 35

When your partner has to go on a trip, hide a small gift for her in the corner of her suitcase. She will find out when she arrives at her destination.

## IDEA # 36

To celebrate the anniversary of your meeting, buy 2 champagne flutes and have them engraved with your names and date, for example: Mal & Kate. May 7, 2002.

Go to the restaurant where you have a reservation and ask the waiter to have your champagne served in these special glasses. This will be a nice surprise and a nice souvenir in your glassware set.

## IDEA # 37

For your partner's birthday, buy 24 red roses. Meet her in front of a store, in a mall for example. Be the first to arrive at the meeting place and make sure she can't see you when she arrives. Your girlfriend has arrived and is waiting for you.

Ask the first person who walks by if they would do you a favor. Give them a rose, show them your partner, and ask them to hand over the rose and say "Happy Birthday Meagan." Do the same with eleven other people. Choose people of different looks and ages. Ideally, the last rose should be given by a child, even if accompanied by parents.

After the twelve roses have been given to her, you can step up and give her your remaining twelve roses.

## IDEA # 38

Always listen carefully when your partner talks about her memories and take note of the information you hear. For example, when your friend tells you about her favorite ice cream that she could only find in this or that store when she was a child.

For a special occasion, choose something from your list that your partner has told you about and find it, it will make him happy for example eating an ice cream from his childhood store.

## IDEA # 39

Take photos of the two of you in different places, add tickets from places you visited together and some trinkets or souvenirs.

Take all these items and have a professional do a three-dimensional art montage on them. If not, do it yourself.

## IDEA # 40

Buy a small decorated wooden box. Find an "old" key and put it in the box. Then have it engraved on a gold plaque: the key to my heart.

Attach the tag to the inside of the box so that the message can be read when the box is opened.

## IDEA # 41

Buy a small tree with your partner and plant it in a place you like.

Every year on your birthday, have a glass of champagne by your tree and see how your love and your tree have grown.

## IDEA # 42

If you shower early in the morning, you may have noticed that the bathroom mirror is still fogged up. Write a message like "Pete loves Kathy" in the fog. This also works on your car windshield in cold weather.

## IDEA # 43

Here is an original gift: give your partner's name to a star. Many agencies allow people to give their name to a star and you receive an official document to authenticate this act.

## IDEA # 44

Find a comic book that tells a story similar to something that happened to you and your partner. For example, if you worked at the same company, look at the adventures of Gaston Lagaffe to see if you can find any similarities to your story.

If this is the case, photocopy the page in question and enlarge it, then put a blank space in the text of the original comic strip.

Replace the original text with an adaptation of your story and make a photocopy of the modified comic strip again to give it an original look.

You can even go so far as to laminate the resulting document before giving it to your partner.

## IDEA # 45

While on vacation with your partner, plan to get up very early one morning to watch the sunrise in a romantic location.

This may seem difficult to implement, but in the end it's really worth doing at least once: witnessing the birth of a new day together is a truly special moment to share with your partner.

## IDEA # 46

If you have a hot tub in your bathroom or hotel room, create a romantic atmosphere by lighting candles around it and placing some rose petals on the surface of the water.

While your partner is relaxing in the bathtub, serve her champagne and chocolate before joining her.

## IDEA # 47

Create "Love Vouchers" that your partner can exchange for "Romantic Gestures".

For example, you can make a coupon that says: This coupon entitles you to: One relaxing foot massage, valid until 07/08/2045

## IDEA # 48

On a warm summer evening, have a picnic in your backyard. Unroll the tablecloth on the ground and eat some sandwiches, fruit... and drink some champagne.

When you're done, you can lie on the ground and admire the stars hand in hand.

## IDEA # 49

Next time it's raining really hard, go for a walk with your partner.

Forget your umbrella. Run through the streets, jump over puddles and get completely soaked.

Lift your partner up, spin her around and kiss her in the rain. Taste the water running down her face and hold her close.

When you get home, take a nice shower and then share a hot drink, preferably in front of the fireplace.

## IDEA # 50

Plan a surprise hot air balloon ride. When you're in the air, treat your partner to a glass of champagne.

## IDEA # 51

When your friend is sitting at a table or desk, gently approach her from behind and massage her shoulders, neck and head.

Finish with a tender kiss on the neck.

**IDEA # 52**

On a normal day, place an ad in the newspaper that says, for example:

Amanda dear, with you by my side, it's Valentine's Day every day. Thank you for being you. I love you. Graham

**IDEA # 53**

Buy a book that you and your partner want to read. Read it all every night in bed, out loud, changing readers with each chapter.

This is an excellent alternative to TV nights.

**IDEA # 54**

While your partner is taking a shower or bath, take her robe and put it in the dryer or on a radiator. When she's done, wrap her in this warm coat.

**IDEA # 55**

Photocopy your hand and fax the copy to your partner with a message that says, "Can I have your hand?"

**IDEA # 56**

Next time you order a pizza, ask for a heart-shaped pizza. The delivery will be a pleasant surprise.

## IDEA # 57

Buy a box of chocolates. Carefully cut out one side of the box so you can put a love note inside. Close the box and give it to your partner.

## IDEA # 58

Rent a tandem bike and go for a ride with your partner. At the end of the ride, have a picnic in the park.

## IDEA # 59

If you are on a business trip, write an account of your day for your partner. For example, "6am: I just woke up and I'm thinking about you. I want you to be here with me. I better go get ready for work on time.

7.00: I'm on the train. It's crowded: it feels like there are zombies. I miss you…

8:30: I just saw my schedule, it's going to be a big day.

9:30: I'm trying to focus on the sales chart for the month but all I can think about is getting lost in your eyes.

…

6:30 pm: Phew, the day is finally over. I count the hours until our meeting.

Send her the report in the mail. This is a great way to show her how much she means to you and how much you miss her when you're not together.

## IDEA # 60

Ask your partner's family what their favorite book was when they were a child.

Buy her a copy of this book and read it to her at night before she goes to sleep.

## IDEA # 61

Send an email to your partner with a story. You can start with:

Chapter 1: "This is the story of Pete and Kate who met at a friend's party on a beautiful summer night...".

Email can continue to develop the beginning of this story, either by telling the truth or by turning that truth into a love story.

End your email with, "and now it's your turn to write chapter two..."

## IDEA # 62

Buy a kite and fly it together on a windy day.

If you can afford it, choose a large model that you can control by joining forces. It's even more fun.

## IDEA # 63

If you feel like going out to dinner with your partner, propose a "surprise dinner". Here's how to do it:

Start the stopwatch on your watch and give yourself 20 minutes. Then ask your friend to choose a number between 5 and 10. Let's say he chose 7.

Give her a coin and tell her that at every 7th intersection on her way, she must toss the coin in the air. If the coin falls heads up, you will turn left. If it lands on its tail side, turn right.

When you've reached 20 minutes, you can simply look for the restaurant closest to where you arrived.

It's a fun game to liven up an outing and discover new places to eat.

**IDEA # 64**

When you both need to go out, grab your camera and wait for your partner to be ready.

When she appears, pretend you're a professional photographer and take lots of pictures with your flash on. While you're taking pictures, bombard her with questions as if she were a famous actress and you were looking for a scoop for your newspaper.

You'll keep him entertained and your photos will be there to remind you.

**IDEA # 65**

If your partner is sick at home, take a day off work to care for her.

Rent videos, make her some nice soup, cover her with a warm blanket and stay with her.

**IDEA # 66**

Over a meal, ask your partner to tell you about something they've always wanted to do.

Next, write down this information so you don't forget it and make the dream come true. For example, if she has always wanted to swim with dolphins, find a water park where this is possible and surprise her.

## IDEA # 67

Rent a romantic movie. Buy popcorn, champagne, strawberries and chocolate. Get ready for a fun night out....

## IDEA # 68

Go to the drive-in to see a movie, but instead of sitting in the car, lay your picnic tablecloth out on the floor. Light a candle and buy some popcorn. Wrap your arms around your partner's shoulders and enjoy the movie.

## IDEA # 69

Create a personalized magazine cover for your partner. To do this, find a beautiful photo of her and a copy of a popular magazine.

Using an editing program or typography, create your magazine cover with the title:

"The 30 Most Beautiful Women of 2005" and your partner in the front page photo.

After pasting this cover on a real magazine, ask your newsagent to put your magazine in a prominent position on her shelf when your friend should arrive. When she arrives, look at the magazines together and have her discover "her" front page.

## IDEA # 70

Fill the trunk of your car with helium balloons. Go somewhere romantic, preferably on top of a hill, for a walk.

Get out of the car and act like you are ready to start the race. At this point, make sure your friend is closer to the car than you are and send her the keys and ask her to get your jumper from the trunk.

When she opens the trunk, all the balloons will fly away except one that you will have tied to the car and on which she can read "I love you".

## IDEA # 71

For a special occasion, have 2 white t-shirts printed with a red heart and the word "LOVE".

To make it very original, half of the heart and the letters "LO" should be printed on the left side of the first shirt and the other half of the heart and the letters "VE" on the right side of the second shirt.

When you walk side by side down the street, the heart will be complete and the message revealed.

## IDEA # 72

On a hot summer day, buy two big water guns and take them with you to the beach.

Fill them out and send one to your friend. The fight can begin.

## IDEA # 73

Share your food with your partner. When you eat a good dish, put a fork in his mouth and tell him, "You have to try this."

This way of sharing everything will make you even closer to your friend and strengthen your relationship.

## IDEA # 74

Don't be afraid to compliment your partner in public. If you're in the middle of a cooking discussion, for example, you can slip in the "Kate makes the best roast in the world" conversation. Shake her hand tightly as you talk about her.

## IDEA # 75

Plan a special day off for yourself. Start with breakfast in bed, go for a walk, go shopping, take a break at a tea room in the afternoon and finish with a romantic dinner at a restaurant.

## IDEA # 76

Buy a "gift certificate" for a facial from the beautician and give it to her with the message, "Voucher for a special treatment for a special person."

## IDEA # 77

Even if you come home after only buying milk, act like you've had an incredible adventure.

Say something like "I was almost there when the snow started falling. The wolves wouldn't n let me in, so I had to fight them...". Then hug your partner like a huge bear.

## IDEA # 78

Send a thank you note to your partner. For example, a note to thank your partner:

Dear Becky, Being with you makes a big difference, I really appreciate your help and love. Tim

## IDEA # 79

If you have children, have their grandparents take care of them for the weekend.

On Friday night, tell your partner that the weekend is yours and reveal all the things you have planned just for the two of you.

## IDEA # 80

Give your partner a magic box. Each month, put a new little gift inside for their enjoyment.

## IDEA # 81

Find your partner's favorite hobby and choose a gift that is truly useful for that activity.

The more specialized the gift, the greater its impact.

Don't hesitate to use all means at your disposal to get information (family, friends, Internet...).

## IDEA # 82

Meet at the masquerade ball. Send an invitation to your partner asking them to meet you dressed in a specific place at 9:00 pm.

Put on your mask and when you get to her, don't say a word. Take her by the hand and lead her onto the dance floor.

## IDEA # 83

On Thursday, ask your partner to pack her suitcase for the weekend. Tell her that she will need comfortable clothes and walking shoes but don't tell her about your destination.

On Friday night, meet her after work and accompany her to a quiet hotel in the countryside where you will spend a romantic and relaxing weekend.

## IDEA # 84

One evening, when you are both home peacefully, take a piece of paper and draw a crystal ball on it.

Ask your partner to look into the crystal ball and tell you what she sees for the two of you in 5 years.

Do the same and discuss your plans and future together.

## IDEA # 85

Come up with a sweet nickname for your partner. It could be something her parents called her when she was little, or it could be something just between the two of you.

## IDEA # 86

If you have a knack for music, write a love song for your partner. Call it, for example, "Song for Natacha."

Have the sheet music printed, a real-looking cover, add a photo of it, and record the song on a CD.

Put everything in a gift bag and give him "his" CD.

## IDEA # 87

Take your partner to a special destination after blindfolding them.

Try to give her a real and unpredictable surprise, like a table set for a meal on top of a hill, or dinner on a boat from another era. It's important that what you've prepared gives her a shock when she removes the blindfold.

## IDEA # 88

Have a big pillow fight. Buy 2 pillows filled with feathers. Make a few tears in the pillows so the feathers fly out and spread everywhere at the height of the fight.

## IDEA # 89

Go for a late afternoon walk away from the city into the countryside. When the sun goes down, build a big fire with the dead wood you gathered together. Sit by the fire and watch the embers fly away into the night.

## IDEA # 90

If your partner uses a computer, take a picture of the two of you and use it as your desktop wallpaper. To do this with Windows, just right click on the image and go to "Set as Desktop Wallpaper".

## IDEA # 91

If you have artistic talent, take drawing lessons, practice until you can get your partner to pose for you.

## IDEA # 92

Take your partner to a festival. Depending on your taste, you can try it out:

1) Jazz Festival

2) Music Festival

3) Festival of culinary specialties

4) Wine Festival

## IDEA # 93

Make a time travel video. Film yourself side by side on the couch. Start the film by saying, "It's June 19, 2005. We decided to make this video to watch on our 25th wedding anniversary.

Then take turns talking to the camera and telling how you feel about your partner, why you love them, and what your plans are. When you're done, put the footage in a safe deposit box at the bank and by your 25th wedding anniversary, you can go back in time to remember everything you shared.

### IDEA # 94

If you're in a secluded spot near a beach or lake and the weather is warm, improvise a swim with your partner, even if you forgot your swimsuits!

### IDEA # 95

This is a great idea if you are away from your partner for a few days. It requires a bit of preparation but it's worth it. Get in the habit of chatting with her on the internet at the same time every night while she is away. Book your ticket to meet her without telling her you're coming to see her.

At the usual time of your online meeting, ask one of your friends to take your place behind the screen using your personal codes. In the meantime, wait behind your friend's door. Call your friend from your cell phone and ask them to text "I miss you so much, I would give anything to be near you and knock on your door."

As soon as they tell you they've sent the message, knock on the door!

### IDEA # 96

Buy your friend a gold fish in an aquarium and give it to her with a card that says, "Of all the fish in the sea, you are my favorite."

### IDEA # 97

When you're both in the car, early in the morning or at sunset, put a CD in your car stereo that contains nature sounds and listen to it on the road while holding hands with your partner.

## IDEA # 98

The day before your partner's birthday, buy helium balloons, flowers and garlands and hide them in a closet. As soon as your partner is asleep, hang the garlands in the bedroom, release the balloons and scatter the flowers around the bed. Waking up your partner on his birthday will be memorable.

## IDEA # 99

Spend a quiet afternoon with your partner at your local library, browse the shelves, take your time, and sit back in the armchairs to start reading.

## IDEA # 100

If you can afford it, rent a convertible sports car for the weekend. Treat your partner to a long white scarf and sunglasses. Take a walk on the beach with the top down.

## IDEA # 101

Serve breakfast in bed to your partner. You can try:

1) Heart-Shaped Fried Eggs. You can find the tool you need in the kitchen accessories section.

2) Toast with maple syrup.

3) Cereals

4) Fruit juice

5) A bouquet of flowers

Printed in Great Britain
by Amazon